Shoulder Surgery for RC Pathology, Arthropathy and Tumors

Edited by Dimitrios D. Nikolopoulos and George K. Safos

Published in London, United Kingdom

Shoulder Surgery for RC Pathology, Arthropathy and Tumors
http://dx.doi.org/10.5772/intechopen.98035
Edited by Dimitrios D. Nikolopoulos and George K. Safos

Contributors
Andrew Konopitski, Ajith Malige, Simona Maria Carmignano, Mohammed Hegazy, Ana C. Belzarena, Stephanie D. Zarate, Reuben Gobezie, Yousef Shishani, Brandon J. Erickson, Amhaz Escanlar S., Jorge Mora A., Pino Miguez J., Vladimir Senekovic

First published in London, United Kingdom, 2022 by IntechOpen
IntechOpen is the global imprint of INTECHOPEN LIMITED, registered in England and Wales, registration number: 11086078, 5 Princes Gate Court, London, SW7 2QJ, United Kingdom

British Library Cataloguing-in-Publication Data
A catalogue record for this book is available from the British Library

Additional hard and PDF copies can be obtained from orders@intechopen.com

Shoulder Surgery for RC Pathology, Arthropathy and Tumors
Edited by Dimitrios D. Nikolopoulos and George K. Safos
p. cm.
Print ISBN 978-1-80355-396-2
Online ISBN 978-1-80355-397-9
eBook (PDF) ISBN 978-1-80355-398-6

Meet the editors

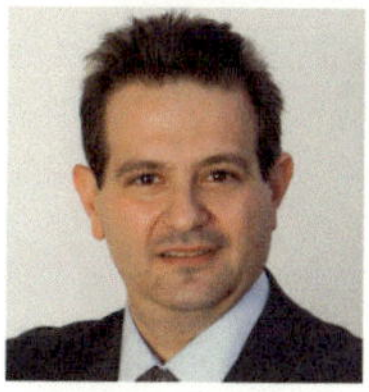

Dr. Dimitrios D. Nikolopoulos, MD, Ph.D., is a sports medicine-specialized orthopedic surgeon and arthroscopist. He focuses on sports injuries, mainly in the shoulder, hip, knee, foot, and ankle pathology. He has performed arthroscopic restoration of hip, knee, and ankle cartilage, as well as treatment and surgical correction of foot disorders. He has published forty-five original scientific articles on the knee (valgus knee) and shoulder surgery (arthroscopic and minimally invasive new techniques), osteoporotic spine and hip fractures, and research into the in vitro environment of bone and cartilage metabolism in prestigious scientific journals in the United States, Europe, and Greece. Dr. Nikolopoulos has more than 240 citations in research projects on the valgus knee and cartilage ankle restoration. He has also presented more than 200 oral and poster presentations internationally.

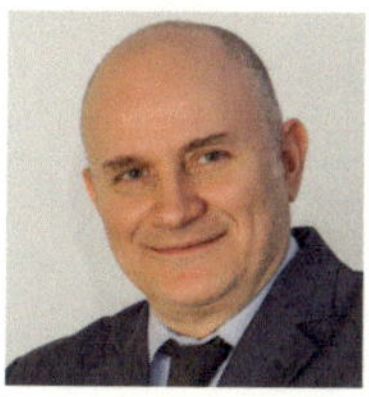

Dr. George K. Safos, MD, specializes in orthopaedic surgery and traumatology with an interest in sports medicine (knee, hip, ankle, elbow, and shoulder arthroscopic surgery) as well as total hip and knee replacement surgery. As a well-published doctor, he now serves as a medical orthopaedic consultant and primary doctor to various athletic teams, and dance groups, as well as for foreign diplomatic missions. He is a graduate of Athens University Medical School and completed his residency in Orthopaedic Surgery and Traumatology at the General Hospital of Asklepeion Voulas, Greece. He then completed two fellowships in the United States at the National Institutes of Health (NIH), Maryland, and the University of Miami Orthopaedics Department. Thereafter, Dr. Safos completed a post-graduate degree in Tissue Banking at the National University of Singapore with a United Nations scholarship.

Contents

Preface

Shoulder injury is a reason for everyday pain in thousands of patients every year. The 340-degree range of movement (ROM) of the shoulder is the cause of many pathologies of the rotator cuff (RC) tendons. Impingement syndrome, rotator cuff rupture, shoulder fractures, and RC arthropathy are painful conditions of the upper extremity resulting in serious discomfort. Shoulder pathology is primarily diagnosed by history and physical examination. The mainstay of treatment involves early identification before the onset of degenerative changes, physical therapy exercises to strengthen the shoulder girdle, and pharmacological interventions to decrease inflammation.

This book describes the pathology, evaluation, and management of shoulder RC pathology and shoulder arthritic changes (arthropathy) and highlights the role of an interprofessional team in the care of patients with these conditions. Open and arthroscopic techniques, especially in the last decade, have changed therapeutic solutions, minimizing the possibility of RC arthropathy and arthritis. In addition, new conservative therapies with stem cells and platelet-rich plasma (PRP) have opened a new field of treatment for shoulder injuries.

Dr. Dimitrios D. Nikolopoulos and Dr. George K. Safos
Central Clinic of Athens,
Athens, Greece

Section 1

Rotator Cuff Pathology

Chapter 1

Review of Ortho-Biologics in Rotator Cuff Repair

Andrew Konopitski and Ajith Malige

Abstract

Rotator cuff repair is one of the most commonly performed surgeries in orthopedics, yet rates of postoperative failure and retear remain relatively high. Poor biology and limited healing potential at the cuff insertion are frequently cited as potential confounders to otherwise technically successful surgeries. Over the past several years, ortho-biologics have been developed in an attempt to augment rotator cuff repairs. The following review will briefly cover normal biomechanics and histology of the rotator cuff and how this is altered in cuff tears, provide an in-depth summary of the available literature on various ortho-biologic agents, outline the limitations of each agent and give an idea on the future of ortho-biologics in rotator cuff.

Keywords: rotator cuff repair, biologics, stem cells, growth factors, platelet rich plasma

1. Introduction

Rotator cuff disease is among the most common causes of shoulder pain and dysfunction in adults. The overall incidence ranges from 87 to 198 cases per 100,000 person-years, with the prevalence only increasing with age [1]. Rotator cuff (RTC) pathology is present in as few as 10% of symptomatic patients under the age of 20 years, but this rate increases precipitously to 63% in patients over 50 years of age [2]. While technology and techniques used in rotator cuff repair (RCR) have evolved, outcomes have generally plateaued. Rates of repair failure continue to range from 20 to 60% and usually occur within the first 15 months of surgery [3]. Furthermore, rotator cuff re-tear has been associated with significant decreases in patient reported outcomes and function [3, 4].

Several factors have been postulated to contribute to the relatively high failure rate of RCR, mostly due to either patient specific versus factors involving surgical technique. Patient related risk factors can be modifiable (smoking, compliance to post-operative protocol, strict blood sugar control) or non-modifiable (RCT size, chronicity, patient age, etc.) [5]. In an effort to improve success after RCR as well as patient outcomes, surgeons have explored the addition of biologic augmentation aimed at addressing each of these obstacles to tendon healing. The goals of this review are as follows:

- Review the normal histology and mechanics of the rotator cuff
- Explain how the repaired cuff differs from the native histological structure

- Introduce several ortho-biologic technologies and their theoretical mechanism of action and how they are surgically implemented
- Review the current literature on each ortho-biologic application
- Provide a brief discussion on future directions in the field of ortho-biologics.

2. Biomechanics and histology of the native and diseased rotator cuff

2.1 Biomechanics

The rotator cuff is a confluence of both static and dynamic stabilizers that work together to maintain the instantaneous center of rotation of the humeral head within the glenoid fossa throughout the arc of shoulder motion [6]. The static stabilizers include four glenohumeral ligaments, the coracohumeral ligament (CHL) and the glenoid labrum. The glenohumeral ligaments are discrete capsuloligamentous bands which become variably tensioned depending on arm position and serve as checkreins to excessive humeral head translation at the extremes of motion [7, 8]. The CHL works in conjunction with the superior glenohumeral ligament (SGHL) to resist inferior humeral head translation with the arm adducted, and the labrum serves not only to deepen the relatively shallow glenoid fossa but also to contribute to the overall negative pressure within the glenohumeral joint [8].

While static stabilizers are instrumental in maintaining normal shoulder biomechanics, they are far less frequently injured than the dynamic stabilizers which fall victim to degenerative changes of age, chronic overuse and acute trauma. The four rotator cuff muscles are the supraspinatus, infraspinatus, teres minor and subscapularis. The supraspinatus originates in the supraspinatus fossa of the scapula and inserts along the superior aspect of the greater tuberosity. Its primary function is to work in conjunction with the deltoid to initiate shoulder abduction and to counteract superior migration of the humeral head [6]. The infraspinatus and teres minor both insert along the posterior aspect of the greater tuberosity and function primarily as external rotators of the shoulder as well as resistors to posterior translation, though the infraspinatus does contribute somewhat to abduction and resistance to superior translation as well [6, 8]. Lastly, the subscapularis originates in the subscapular fossa and inserts broadly along the lesser tuberosity, medial to the bicipital groove where it becomes confluent with the transverse humeral ligament. The subscapularis is a strong internal rotator of the humerus, resists anterior and inferior translation, and provides stability to the biceps tendon [8]. Disruption of any one of these dynamic stabilizers can result in the loss of the physiologic force coupling between the humeral head and the glenoid leading to pain, weakness, reduced active range of motion and eventual degenerative changes.

2.2 Histology

Understanding the histology of the rotator cuff is imperative in order to contextualize the use of biologic adjuncts to improve healing responses. Near their insertion points on the greater tuberosity, the tendons of the supraspinatus and infraspinatus become confluent into one conjoined tendon. The microscopic cross-sectional anatomy of the conjoined tendon has been described as being 5 distinct layers.

Layer 1 is the most superficial layer composed of fibers from the CHL and is rich in blood supply. Layer 2 is composed of large bundles of parallel tendon fibers with arterioles from layer 1 intermixed. Layer 3 has small diameter tendinous bundles which are loosely packed and have a sparse blood supply. Layer 4 is primarily loose connective tissue with collagen bundles, and Layer 5 is continuous with the joint capsule and inserts on the humerus as Sharpey fibers [9]. More simply, the cuff can be thought of as having a bursal side superficially and an articular side abutting the joint capsule. The bursal side has more tensile strength and better vascularity than the joint side, yet it is prone to degenerative tears frequently resulting from impingement whereas joint sided tears often result from acute trauma [10].

The blood supply to the rotator cuff plays an important role in both injury and healing potential. Codman in 1934 first described a "critical zone" of the supraspinatus tendon roughly 1 cm proximal to its insertion on the greater tuberosity which exhibited poor blood supply. A cadaveric study by Determe et al. in 1996 confirmed the presence of this hypovascular zone, and Levy et al. later showed that the presence of this hypovascular zone is exacerbated in impingement [11, 12]. It has therefore been postulated that the critical zone plays a significant role in the development of degenerative rotator cuff tears and may also provide a suboptimal environment for tendon healing after attempted repair.

The tendon-bone interface, known as the enthesis, is the region of the RTC most prone to tears and can be separated into four distinct zones: tendon, nonmineralized fibrocartilage, mineralized fibrocartilage, and bone [13–16]. Healing of rotator cuff tears (RCT) progresses through three overlapping stages. Stage 1 (0–7 days) is characterized as the inflammatory phase. In this stage, damaged tissues release various cytokines which recruit inflammatory cells such as neutrophils, monocytes and fibroblasts. These inflammatory cells release further cytokines, clear cellular debris and promote early angiogenesis. Stage 2 is the repair phase (5–21 days) in which a pro-fibrotic environment causes scar formation primarily composed of type III collagen. Stage 3 is the remodeling phase which can last for up to 8 weeks where type III collagen is steadily converted into type I [17]. Unfortunately, even after complete remodeling, the resulting healed scar at the enthesis fails to reach the same biomechanical strength as the native tendon insertion [13]. This is compounded by the frequent formation of gaps within the repaired tendon which have been shown through post-operative ultrasonographic and MRI studies [18–20]. The aim of ortho-biologic augmentation in RCR is to create an environment which minimizes the amount of type III collagen scar formation and instead

3. Osteoinductive growth factors

The introduction of osteogenic growth factors in RCR is one of the earliest uses of biologic augmentation aimed at improving the healing response. Studies have shown that healing of a repaired cuff tendon to bone is dependent on bony ingrowth. In vitro studies were able to demonstrate improved attachment strength of tendon within bone tunnels with the addition of bone morphogenic proteins (BMPs) [20]. Through immunohistological staining, Würgler-Hauri et al. isolated eight different osteoinductive growth factors (bFGF, BMP-12, BMP-13, BMP-14, COMP, CTGF, PDGF-B, and TGF-β1) which were temporally expressed throughout the 16 week arc of healing [21]. Following this, Rodeo et al. in 2007 were the first to introduce an exogenous osteogenic bone protein extract in vivo in a sheep model. A bovine derived extract contained a mixture of BMP-2, BMP-7, transforming growth factor-β-1-3 (TGF-β1, TGF-β3) and fibroblast growth factor (FGF) which was impregnated into a type I collagen sponge and placed over the repair site. This study demonstrated greater formation of new bone, fibrocartilage, and soft tissue, with a concomitant increase in tendon attachment strength, but less stiffness than repairs treated with the type I collagen sponge carrier alone [20]. An important caveat to this study is that MRI evaluation of the repairs showed consistent gap formation at the repair sites.

3.1 Bone morphogenic proteins

BMPs are part of the TGF-β family and have been identified as growth factors important for new bone formation [22]. In vitro studies of BMP-2 and 7 have demonstrated dose dependent increases in type I collagen production, expression and cellular activity [22, 23]. Further in vitro study of BMP-7 has shown that it can induce differentiation of mesenchymal stem cells into chondrocytes which promotes the regeneration of interfacial cartilage and improves the quality of tendon healing [24]. In both rabbit and rat models, BMP-2 and 7 have demonstrated the ability to enhance new bone formation and tensile strength in repaired tendon insertions [24–26]. Unfortunately, no studies have been published on the use of BMP-2 or 7 in human RCR.

BMP-12 and 13 are thought to be important regulators of fibrocartilage, neotendon, and ligament formation [27]. There are limited in vitro studies of BMP-12 and 13 in the literature, but several in vivo studies have been published. Seeherman et al. in 2008 used human recombinant BMP-12 (rhBMP-12) on a collagen sponge carrier in the sheep model which resulted in higher tensile strength and faster healing times compared to untreated controls [28]. In the rat model, Lamplot et al. administered recombinant adenoviral vectors which caused the upregulation of BMP-13 and found increased biomechanical strength in the healing tendons after 2 weeks [29]. There is one randomized, multicenter study in humans which implanted an absorbable collagen sponge treated with BMP-12. This study did demonstrate safety of BMP-12, but did not evaluate whether there were any clinical, biomechanical or structural improvements with BMP-12 treatment [30].

BMP-14 has been found at the tendon edges on the bursal side of torn rotator cuffs. In conjunction with BMP-13, it has been shown to increase the tensile strength of regenerated tendon [31]. As of yet, no human studies have evaluated the safety or efficacy of BMP-13 or 14 in isolation for RCR.

3.2 Platelet derived growth factors

Platelet derived growth factor (PDGF) includes a family of 5 soluble, dimeric glycoproteins (PDGF-AA, -BB, -CC, -DD, -EE) which are released from alpha granules in platelets. PDGF-BB has been shown to have mitogenic and chemotactic effects on tenocytes, fibroblasts and mesenchymal stems cells and is another important growth factor in tendon healing [32]. One notable point which has been demonstrated with PDGF research is the influence of timing of administration on tendon healing, as not all growth factors are present at equal concentrations throughout the healing process. The normal peak PDGF-BB concentration occurs between 7 and 14 days after surgical repair [31]. In a rat patellar-tendon defect model, there was an increased proliferative response when PDGF-BB was injected on day 3 after surgery, and addition of PDGF-BB on day 7 improved peak load and pyridinoline content after administration of the highest dosage of PDGF [33, 34].

The primary modes of administration for PDGF-BB are by way of suture dip-coated with the growth factor or by being housed within a type I collagen scaffold. PDGF-BB dip-coated suture did show overall improved histological scores in sheep models, but there was no significant increase in ultimate load-to-failure after 6 weeks [32]. Studies measuring the effect of PDGF-BB impregnated collagen scaffolds in rat models have provided heterogeneous results and no study has been conducted in humans [35, 36].

3.3 Transforming growth factor-β

Transforming growth factor-β (TGF-β) is a ubiquitous growth factor which is present throughout all phases of tendon healing and is secreted by all cells participating in the healing response including platelets, lymphycytes, macrophages, endothelial cells and fibroblasts [37]. The three isoforms most closely linked to scar formation and tendon healing are TGF-β1, TGF-β2 and TGF-β3. Initial studies in TGF-β came from information gained through the study of healing fetal tissues. It was found that wound healing in fetal tissue is marked with decreased expression of TGF-β1 and β2 with increased expression of TGF-β3 [38]. These studies in fetal wound healing spawned a plethora of similar explorations of TGF-β as it relates to tendon healing in the rotator cuff. An early study performed by Kim et al. on rat supraspinatus models, neutralizing antibodies were used in conjunction with an osmotic pump to allow for the selective presence of each TGF-β isoform in isolation. They found that type III collagen production was increased in the context of TGF-β1, but were unable to show significant differences in mechanical properties with any of the isoforms [39]. At the same time, Manning et al. used a heparin/fibrin-based delivery system to affect a sustained concentration of TGF-β3 to the supraspinatus tendon of rats. They found significant improvements in tendon healing histologically as well as improved biomechanical strength [38]. Several years later, Yoon et al. again tested the sustained administration of TGF-β, but this time using the TGF-β1 isoform. This study found improved mechanical and histological properties of sustained TGF-β1 delivery on an alginate scaffold compared to a single TGF-β1 injection or suture repair alone in the rabbit models [40]. Most recently, Yoon et al. (2021) again tested a sustained release model of TGF-β1, but this time they developed a porous suture containing the growth factor and tested it on a rat model. They found similar improvements in the biomechanical and histological properties with the porous suture containing TGF-β1 compared to controls [41]. As of yet, no study has evaluated the safety or efficacy of isolated TGF-β biologics in human RCR.

3.4 Basic fibroblast growth factor

Early in vitro studies of basic fibroblast growth factor (bFGF) highlighted the importance of this growth factor in promoting the proliferation of mesenchymal stem cells as well as collagen production [42]. BFGF, specifically FGF-2, causes fibroblasts to produce collagenase and stimulates proliferation of capillary endothelial cells, both of which are necessary for angiogenesis. It also helps to initiate the formation of granulation tissue [34]. In one of the earliest studies investigating bFGF on rotator cuff tissue in mice, Ide et al. combined FGF-2 with a fibrin sealant which was then placed within the greater tuberosity decortication site. They compared the FGF-2 additive to fibrin sealant alone and found that the repair sites were histologically more mature and biomechanically stronger at 2 weeks, but these improvements were not seen at 4 and 6 weeks [43]. Later, Lu et al. loaded bFGF onto a hydroxyapatite coated orthocord suture and found that the addition of bFGF increased tendon thickness, but did not show histological improvements [44].

With the advent of collagen scaffolds (discussed below), in vivo studies of bFGF have greatly expanded. In 2015, Peterson et al. used an FGF-2 impregnated scaffold in the repair of ovine supraspinatus tendons. At 8 weeks they found thicker tendon formation which mimicked native tendon structure, more new bone formation, less gap formation and improved biomechanical properties compared to controls [45]. Tokunaga et al. translated this information to the rabbit model and tested two different concentrations of FGF-2, 3 μg and 30 μg, in a gelatin hydrogel sheet which was inlayed into the greater tuberosity decortication site prior to tendon repair. At 12 weeks both treatment groups demonstrated improved histologic and biomechanical properties compared to controls [46]. Similar improvements in histologic scores and biomechanical strength have now been found with the addition of FGF-2 to chronic RTC tears as well as in the context of platelet-rich plasma (discussed below) [47, 48]. However, while in vivo evidence supporting the use of bFGF in tendon repair appears robust, there is no current evidence addressing the safety or efficacy of bFGF in human RCR.

4. Platelet-rich plasma

Platelet-rich plasma (PRP) has been extensively studied in its use as a stand-alone or adjunctive treatment option for rotator cuff tears, with its use projected to continue to increase in the coming years. This autologous agent is obtained from the patient and centrifuged down in a cost effective manner [49], resulting in a plasma layer that is highly concentrated in platelets (3–5 times higher than in normal blood) [50]. It is then most commonly delivered as an injectable concentration to the desired site. PRP can also be made [17] into a gel state that allows delivery to a specific area with prolonged function [51]. Ersen et al. studied the delivery method of PRP, finding that injectable PRP and absorption from a PRP sponge have similar effects on tendon-bone interface biomechanical properties [52].

There are four types of formulations described: platelet-rich fibrin matrices made from activating autogenous thrombin with the plasma, leukocyte-platelet-rich plasma made by retaining leukocytes while preparing the PRP concentration, platelet rich in growth factors, and an autologous conditioned plasma that is an Arthrex product (Naples, FL, United States) made from a centrifuged solution of autologous blood [53–55]. Regardless of type, PRPs have been theorized to be efficacious in tendon repair due to their myriad of growth factors and cytokines, including transforming growth factor beta (TGF-β), basic fibroblast growth factor (FGF), insulin-like growth factor (IGF-1), vascular endothelial growth factor (VEGF), and platelet rich derived growth factor (PDGF) [56–60].

Proponents of PRP argue that it is an easily harvestable autologous agent with a low-risk profile that offers the potential to deliver high concentrations of beneficial growth factors. Detractors note that the final PRP concentration can be highly variable based on patient biology and the preparation process [61]. When considering their benefit in RCR specifically, in vitro studies have theorized that PRP not only increases tenocyte matrix synthesis and cell proliferation but also can activate existing tenocyte progenitor cells that can aid in tendon regeneration and healing [62–64]. Hoppe et al. theorized that existing fibroblasts showed increased proliferation in the presence of PRP, citing PRP as a beneficial activator in the healing process [65]. Dolkart et al. used a rat model to demonstrate a higher load to failure, better stiffness, and improved histological characteristics in a PRP-augmented RCR [66].

Based on these theorized benefits, PRP has been explored as a stand-alone non-operative treatment option for rotator cuff tears. Kesiburun et al. compared PRP injections to saline injections, finding that there was no difference in pain scores or functional outcomes between the two treatment options [67]. Shams et al. compared subacromial PRP injections to corticosteroid injections, finding that both groups had improved pain scores post-injection. They also found that patients who received PRP injections had more pain relief at 3 months postoperatively but similar pain improvement at 6 months compared to the corticosteroid injection group [68].

Studies exploring PRP as an adjunct during surgical rotator cuff repair are heterogeneous and hard to draw conclusions from due to the variety of patient biology, cuff tear patterns, tendon quality, and repair techniques. Studies have demonstrated the imaging-backed conclusion that PRP injections improve structural healing rates of the injured tendon with decreased failure rates [69]. This is important, especially in younger patients, since this can be associated with improved strength and overhead function. Hurley et al. in their review showed that PRP can reduce the rate of incomplete tendon healing in small to medium sized tears and medium to large sized tears [70]. A few studies have built off of these improvements in tendon healing and have noted improvements in patient satisfaction and pain scores after rotator cuff repairs utilizing PRP [71]. Multiple studies have noted lower re-tear rates after RCR utilizing PRP as well [69, 72, 73].

However, for the most part these improvements in tendon healing have not resulted in sustained clinical improvements, as most studies detail a lack of differences long-term in patients who undergo rotator cuff repair with PRP using an adjunct versus those who undergo a repair in isolation [74–76]. Charousset et al. found no difference in outcomes, both functional and radiographic, or re-tear rates between repairs completed utilizing leukocyte-rich PRP and those without [77]. Rodeo et al. in their randomized controlled trial reported no difference in tendon healing or functional improvement after RCR utilizing platelet rich PRP versus repairs without an adjunct. Interestingly, they did report that using this PRP came with a 5.8 higher likelihood of tendon-bone healing failure at 12 weeks compared to repairs without this adjunct [78]. Ruiz-Moneo et al. reported similar improvements in functional outcomes, patient satisfaction, and tendon healing after RCR utilizing PRP versus repair without it [79]. These similarities between groups remained in studies that looked at 10-year outcomes after RCR utilizing PRP versus RCR alone [80].

5. Stem cells

The use of stem cells to enhance tendon healing responses is a fairly new and quickly evolving field. It has become evident that tendon healing is a complex process that involves the overlapping of a multitude of growth factors and cell types. Targeting pluripotent stem cells to RCR sites can theoretically prompt the cells to differentiate into the tenocyte lineage, thus allowing for the production of all the required growth factors and machinery to create a more robust repair that mimics the native tendon. The following sections will focus on different sources for stem cells and will summarize the evidence available for each in the context of RCR.

5.1 Bone marrow-derived mesenchymal stem cells

Mesenchymal stem cells are pluripotent cells which can differentiate into any tissue of mesenchymal embryologic origin including muscle, fat, bone and tendon. This, along with the relative ease with which the cells can be obtained via bone marrow aspirate, make bone marrow-derived mesenchymal stem cells (BMSC) attractive candidates for biologic augmentation in RCR.

In vivo studies of BMSCs have been flooding the literature over the last 10–15 years and have utilized several different animal models as well as delivery methods. A summary of the literature can be found in **Table 1**. Overall, in vivo data supporting the use of BMSC in isolation or in combination with other factors such as PRP or demineralized bone matrix is strong. It has been shown repeatedly that histology of repaired tendon in the context of BMSC tends to closely align with native tendon structure and biomechanical strength has been shown to improve in concert with this data [83–87].

5.2 Adipose-derived stem cells

Adipose-derived stem cells (ADSC) have been a more recent focus of investigation than BMSCs, but have similarly strong in vivo data supporting their use. ADSCs share a similar advantage to BMSCs in that they are fairly easily harvested and have significant pluripotent cell potential [98]. The most commonly cited method for purification of ADSCs is the protocol outlined by Zuk et al. in a series of eight steps: obtain adipose tissue by liposuction, wash raw lipoaspirate, enzymatically digest lipoaspirate, centrifugal separation, lyse contaminating red blood cells, filter, incubate, and final wash to remove residual red blood cells [98, 99].

A summary of the available evidence for the use of ADSCs is found in **Table 1**, but only three of these studies were based on human trials. Kim et al. in 2017 injected ADSC along with a fibrin glue at the conclusion of surgical repair. At one year, the patients treated with ADSC and fibrin glue did have a significantly lower retear rate, though this did not translate into improved pain or functional scores compared to control [100]. The following year Jo et al. published two studies in which they injected ADSCs directly into partial RCTs. In the first of the two studies, patients were given either a low, mid or high concentration of ADSC in order to establish safety and tolerability. After this, a second study was conducted where all patients received the high concentration injection. In both studies, patients exhibited improved pain and functional scores as well as near complete RCT healing on repeat MRI evaluation at 2 years [101, 102]. While the number of patients included in this study was relatively small, the results show promise for future applications.

5.3 Umbilical cord blood-derived mesenchymal stem cells

Of the various tissues containing mesenchymal stem cells, human umbilical cord blood-derived MSCs (UCB-MSC) have theoretical benefits over other tissue derivatives including: (1) the ability to home in on injured tissue, (2) low immunogenicity, (3) multidirectional differentiation, (4) extensive secretion profiles, (5) ability to be produced commercially in large quantities with homogenous quality and (6) allogenic UCB-MSCs are not prone to degenerative impairments of age seen with autologous MSCs [95].

First author, year	Cell type	Vehicle	Animal model	Major findings
Gulotta, 2009 [81]	BMSC	Fibrin	Rat RCT	No change in histology or biomechanics at 2 or 4 weeks
Gulotta, 2011 [82]	BMSC + Scleraxis	Fibrin	Rat RCT	Improved histology and biomechanical strength at 4 weeks
Yokoya, 2012 [83]	BMSC	PGA sheet	Rabbit RCT	Improved histology and biomechanical strength at 8 weeks
Hernigou, 2014 [84]	BMSC	Injection	Human RCT	Improved healing rates by US/MRI with lower rates of retear at 10 years
Degan, 2016 [85]	BMSC	Fibrin	Rat RCT	Early histoligic and biomechanical improvement at 2 weeks, no significance at 4 weeks
Thangarajah, 2017 [86]	BMSC	DBM	Chronic rat RCT	Enhanced bone mineral density at enthesis at 6 weeks
Han, 2019 [87]	BMSC + PRP	Injection	Rat RCT	Improved histology and biomechanical strength at 8 and weeks
Oh, 2014 [88]	ADSC	Injection	Rabbit RCT	Improved histology and biomechanical strength at 6 weeks
Mora, 2014 [89]	ADSC	Collagen Scaffold	Rat RCT	Decreased inflammation, no change in biomechanical properties
Lipner, 2015 [90]	ADSC + BMP2	Nanofiber scaffold	Rat RCT	Decreased mechanical properties, no change in bone mineral density
Chen, 2015 [91]	ADSC	Injection	Rat RCT	Initially improved histology and biomechanical strength at 7 days, no significant difference at 28 days
Rothrauff, 2019 [92]	ADSC + TGF-β3	Fibrin, GelMA	Rat RCT	ADSC in isolation provided greatest improvement in bone mineral density over TGF-β3 additive
Wang, 2019 [93]	ADSC exosomes	Injection	Rat RCT	Improved histology and biomechanical strength at 16 weeks
Park, 2015 [94]	UCB-MSC	Injection	Rabbit RCT	Partial thickness tendon healing with type I collagen
Kwon, 2018 [95]	UCB-MSC + PDRN	Injection	Rabbit RTC	Improved histological and functional outcomes
Kwon, 2018 [96]	UCB-MSC + PDRN	Injection	Rabbit RTC	No significant differences with treatment
Kwon, 2018 [97]	UCB-MSC	Scaffold	Rabbit RTC	Improved histological and functional outcomes

BMSC—bone marrow-derived stem cells, RCT—rotator cuff tear, PGA—polyglycolic acid, PRP—platelet rich plasma, ADSC—Adipose-derived stem cells, BMP2—bone morphogenic protein 2, TGF-β3—transforming growth factor beta 3, UCB-MSC—umbilical cord blood-derived mesenchymal stem cell, PDRN—polydeoxyribonucleotudes.

Table 1.
Summary of studies conducted using mesenchymal stem cell derivatives.

Thus far, all published data on UCB-MSCs has been conducted on animal models that undergo a simulated RCT followed by the later injection of UCB-MSCs under ultrasound guidance with no attempt at underlying repair. A summary of the available data can be found in **Table 1**. While all studies have shown the ability to produce at least partial thickness healing with a high concentration of type I collagen, further investigation is needed to determine the utility of UCB-MSCs in the context of RCR. It should also be noted that all the available literature regarding UCB-MSC has been published solely out of Catholic University of Daegu School of Medicine in South Korea.

5.4 Subacromial bursa-derived cells

Perhaps the most recent tissue type to be harvested for stem cells is subacromial bursa tissue. The potential for subacromial bursal tissue to supply mesenchymal stem cells was first described in a protocol outlined by Lhee et al. where human tissue was obtained, treated with a collagenase to isolate cells, then serially cultured. The resulting cell lines were then subject to immunohistochemical staining to confirm their mesenchymal potential [103]. This process was later refined by Morikawa et al. in an effort to identify an effective, nonenzymatic method for maximizing the yield of subacromial bursa-derived nucleated cells (SBDC). They found that a mechanical chopping method of tissue processing led to similar yields of SBDC which could easily be implanted during surgery [104]. Morikawa et al. also conducted an in vitro study in an effort to compare SBDC to BMSC (discussed above) and found that SBDC possessed significantly increased differentiation ability and gene expression over time compared to BMSC [105]. This data has been further substantiated by the work of Meunch et al. and Landry et al. [106, 107].

Thus far, no in vivo or human trials investigating SBDCs have been published. Freislederer et al. did publish a technique in which subacromial bursal tissue from the lateral subdeltoid region is used to overlay the RCR and sutured in place, but no long-term results from this technique have been reported [108].

6. Scaffolding devices

Biomaterials that are used as a scaffold during rotator cuff repair should fulfill the following four criteria: (1) they should withstand the stresses placed at the bone-tendon interface by mimicking the biomechanical properties of native tissue (2) the physical structure should closely mimic fibrocartilage 3.) the material should both be biodegradable and lack side effects during degradation 4.) the biomaterial should be capable of being used in multiple settings and have multiple functions [22]. Furthermore, pore diameter, especially in porous scaffolds, is important to consider, as smaller pores are inefficient and larger pores can compromise the scaffold's mechanical properties [109].

Biological, or natural, scaffolds have been formed from human, equine, porcine, and bovine sources. All the non-collagen components are processed out while the collagen 1-predominant structure is kept in order to maintain its biomechanical properties [110]. Other scaffolds designed from natural polymers include silk, fibrin, and polysaccharide based augments [111]. Silk scaffolds in particular have been greatly explored due to its biodegradable and biocompatible properties. They have been theorized to both be reliable augments as well as a scaffold for stem cell delivery to the repair site [112, 113].

Synthetic scaffolds trade out the ability to have better biomechanical properties compared to natural scaffolds for limited biocompatibility when used *in vivo*.

These scaffolds are theoretically more versatile in their tailoring and utilization as rotator cuff repair augments as well, representing a possibly reproducible source that can deliver growth factors and stimulate tendon healing with low immunogenicity. However, the lack of biomechanical or clinical superiority of these scaffolds compared to natural scaffolds has stifled much enthusiasm towards exploring these structures in rotator cuff repairs [111, 114, 115].

Extracellular matrices have been recently developed as a scaffold patch to support both cell attachment and matrix formation, aiding in tendon healing after rotator cuff repair [116]. These patches have been theorized to help augment repairs either by acting as a load-sharing device that reduces strain across the repair site or by acting as a scaffold to support cell attachment, matrix synthesis, and new tissue formation [117]. Data on the efficacy of this augment is limited but promising. Bokor et al. utilized a collagen patch augmentation and found new tissue formation in all patients by 3 months after repair and a nearly normal-looking rotator cuff tendon by 12 months [118].

Nanomaterial scaffolds are a more recently developed and utilized polymer that have had promising results. They have a high surface area to volume ratio and can be easily altered for their intended use. They have had promising *in vitro*, animal, and clinical studies showing the potential to be used regularly to improve results due to their ability to be a platform for nanotopography-mediated cell response, the incorporation of stem cells, and the housing and delivery of active growth factors [119–123]. Based on the structure and biomolecular basis of these scaffolds, they have been shown to aid in cell proliferation [124], osteogenic differentiation [125], osteogenesis [126], and improving the biomechanical strength [127] of the healing tendon.

Hydrogel scaffolds have also been explored as useful, biocompatible scaffolds. Hydrogels are gelatinous viscoelastic structures that can be utilized in various forms while augmenting rotator cuff repairs. They have been loaded with exogenous biomolecules, including platelet-derived growth factor [35] and bone morphogenic protein (BMP) [26], as well as delivered directly *in vivo* in combination with progenitor cells and BMP and allowed to polymerize [128]. Both utilizations yielded a bone-tendon interface that showed greater collagen fiber orientation, improved biomechanical properties, and higher ultimate failure loads.

7. Vesicular phospholipid gels

Vesicular phospholipid gels (VPGs) are lecithin and aqueous buffer solutions that allow for the non-toxic and safe prolonged release of growth factors to a specific location. These products are easy to produce and easy to deliver to a desired location with minimal systemic effects. This product can theoretically house and deliver any product that can help improve tendon healing [129, 130]. Buchmann et al. showed that VPGs filled with granulocyte colony-stimulating factor improved load-to-failure ratio and improved collagen I/III ratios when combined with rotator cuff repairs compared with repairs done without VPGs [129].

8. Matrix metalloproteinase inhibitors

Matrix metalloproteinases (MMPs) are a group of enzymes belonging to a family of 24 zinc-dependent endopeptidases that exist as inactive proenzymes and become activated after proteolysis secondary to physiologic or pathologic conditions. Once active, they break down extracellular matrix components and have been found in high concentrations with acute RCTs, especially MMP-13 [22, 131, 132]. It has therefore been hypothesized that inhibiting local MMP activity in RCR will lead to a more robust healing response. Bedi et al. conducted a rat based study in which three treatment groups were given 130 mg/kg oral doxycycline, a known MMP synthesis inhibitor, at different time frames. Group 1 was treated in the immediate postoperative period, group 2 was given oral doxycycline starting 5 days postop, and group 3 began doxycycline treatment 14 days postoperatively. Groups 1 and 2 exhibited improved histologic healing and load to failure, while group 3 demonstrated no such benefit [133]. The same group of researchers conducted a follow-up study in a rat model in which alpha-2-macroglobuline (A2M) was locally applied to the RCR intraoperatively. While the repair sites did show improved histologic collagen organization, they failed to demonstrate biomechanical improvements [134].

Studies looking at the effects of MMP inhibition in RCR are limited in both scope and number, but preliminary in vivo studies have provided promise for future investigation.

9. Future directions

The most recent research has veered away from utilizing exogenous agents and towards utilizing intrinsic progenitor cells, or the "stem cell niche." It is theorized that while most of these cells are quiescent at baseline, they are stimulated during tissue injury and repair, and this property can be utilized during RCR. This includes sources such as previscular mesenchymal stem cells [135], subacromial bursa [136], and umbilical cord blood [95] among others. Furthermore, continued work is necessary to try to maximize the localization of stem cell treatments and avoid any systemic effects, side effects, or possible cellular mutations that can adversely affect the patient [22]. Finally, most adjuncts have been studied in isolation. The combination of one or more of the already discussed adjuncts could help achieve results that are more efficacious than any adjunct used in isolation.

Outside of the utilization of indogenous agents, gene therapy and gene editing has also been hypothesized as a possible target in helping to improve the biologic activity of progenitor cell lineages. The exosomes of mesenchymal stem cells have recently been extracted and studied as a possible adjunct. It is hypothesized that M2 macrophage-derived exosomes contain proteins and RNA that can stimulate tendon healing without triggering an immune rejection response; however, further research is necessary to truly know if they have a beneficial role in tendon healing and whether any benefit will translate to improved clinical outcomes [137, 138]. The use of augmented sutures and anchors should also continue to be explored [139]. The study of biomaterials that re-create the bone-tendon interface and can augment tendon repair have also been of interest recently and should continue to be explored [140]. Finally, nanotechnology has only been recently explored as a possible adjunct in aiding RCR success and can continue to be a topic of exploration [141].

Conflict of interest

The authors declare no conflict of interest.

Author details

Andrew Konopitski* and Ajith Malige
St. Luke's University Health Network, Bethlehem, United States

*Address all correspondence to: andrew.konopitski@gmail.com

References

[1] White JJE, Titchener AG, Fakis A, Tambe AA, Hubbard RB, Clark DI. An epidemiological study of rotator cuff pathology using the health improvement network database. Bone & Joint Journal. 2014;**96-B**(3):350-353

[2] Teunis T, Lubberts B, Reilly BT, Ring D. A systematic review and pooled analysis of the prevalence of rotator cuff disease with increasing age. Journal of Shoulder and Elbow Surgery. 2014;**23**(12):1913-1921

[3] Chona DV, Lakomkin N, Lott A, Workman AD, Henry AC, Kuntz AF, et al. The timing of retears after arthroscopic rotator cuff repair. Journal of Shoulder and Elbow Surgery. 2017;**26**(11):2054-2059

[4] Garcia GH, Liu JN, Degen RM, Johnson CC, Wong AC, Dines DM, et al. Erratum to "higher critical shoulder angle increases the risk of retear after rotator cuff repair" [J shoulder elbow Surg 2017;26:241-245]. Journal of Shoulder and Elbow Surgery. 2017;**26**(4):732

[5] Menon RS, Wragg NM, Wilson SL. Rotator cuff repair augmentation using Osteoinductive growth factors. SN Comprehensive Clinical Medicine. 2019;**1**:267-276. DOI: 10.1007/s42399-019-0041-z

[6] Carbone S, Gumina S. Rotator cuff biomechanics. Rotator Cuff Tear. 2017;**1**:45-51. DOI: 10.1007/978-3-319-33355-7_3

[7] Warner JJP, Caborn DNM, Berger R, Fu FH, Seel M. Dynamic capsuloligamentous anatomy of the glenohumeral joint. Journal of Shoulder and Elbow Surgery. 1993;**2**:115-133. DOI: 10.1016/s1058-2746(09)80048-7

[8] Lugo R, Kung P, Ma CB. Shoulder biomechanics. European Journal of Radiology. 2008;**68**(1):16-24

[9] Clark JM, Harryman DT 2nd. Tendons, ligaments, and capsule of the rotator cuff. Gross and microscopic anatomy. The Journal of Bone and Joint Surgery. American Volume. 1992;**74**(5):713-725

[10] Nakajima T, Rokuuma N, Hamada K, Tomatsu T, Fukuda H. Histologic and biomechanical characteristics of the supraspinatus tendon: Reference to rotator cuff tearing. Journal of Shoulder and Elbow Surgery. 1994;**3**:79-87. DOI: 10.1016/s1058-2746(09)80114-6

[11] Determe D, Rongières M, Kany J, Glasson JM, Bellumore Y, Mansat M, et al. Anatomic study of the tendinous rotator cuff of the shoulder. Surgical and Radiologic Anatomy. 1996;**18**:195-200. DOI: 10.1007/bf02346127

[12] Levy O, Relwani J, Zaman T, Even T, Venkateswaran B, Copeland S. Measurement of blood flow in the rotator cuff using laser Doppler flowmetry. Journal of Bone and Joint Surgery. British Volume (London). 2008;**90**(7):893-898

[13] Cheung EV, Silverio L, Sperling JW. Strategies in biologic augmentation of rotator cuff repair: A review. Clinical Orthopaedics and Related Research. 2010;**468**(6):1476-1484

[14] Galatz LM, Sandell LJ, Rothermich SY, Das R, Mastny A, Havlioglu N, et al. Characteristics of the rat supraspinatus tendon during tendon-to-bone healing after acute injury. Journal of Orthopaedic Research. 2006;**24**(3):541-550

[15] Gerber C, Schneeberger AG, Perren SM, Nyffeler RW. Experimental

rotator cuff repair. A preliminary study. The Journal of Bone and Joint Surgery. American Volume. 1999;**81**(9):1281-1290

[16] Thomopoulos S, Hattersley G, Rosen V, Mertens M, Galatz L, Williams GR, et al. The localized expression of extracellular matrix components in healing tendon insertion sites: An in situ hybridization study. Journal of Orthopaedic Research. 2002;**20**:454-463. DOI: 10.1016/s0736-0266(01)00144-9

[17] Zumstein M-A, Lädermann A, Raniga S, Schär M-O. The biology of rotator cuff healing. Orthopaedics & Traumatology, Surgery & Research. 2017;**103**(1):S1-S10

[18] Harryman DT 2nd, Mack LA, Wang KY, Jackins SE, Richardson ML, Matsen FA 3rd. Repairs of the rotator cuff. Correlation of functional results with integrity of the cuff. The Journal of Bone and Joint Surgery. American Volume. 1991;**73**(7):982-989

[19] Galatz LM, Ball CM, Teefey SA, Middleton WD, Yamaguchi K. The outcome and repair integrity of completely arthroscopically repaired large and massive rotator cuff tears. The Journal of Bone and Joint Surgery. American Volume. 2004;**86**(2):219-224

[20] Rodeo SA, Potter HG, Kawamura S, Turner AS, Kim HJ, Atkinson BL. Biologic augmentation of rotator cuff tendon-healing with use of a mixture of osteoinductive growth factors. The Journal of Bone and Joint Surgery. American Volume. 2007;**89**(11):2485-2497

[21] Würgler-Hauri CC, Dourte LM, Baradet TC, Williams GR, Soslowsky LJ. Temporal expression of 8 growth factors in tendon-to-bone healing in a rat supraspinatus model. Journal of Shoulder and Elbow Surgery. 2007;**16**:S198-S203. DOI: 10.1016/j.jse.2007.04.003

[22] Patel S, Gualtieri AP, Lu HH, Levine WN. Advances in biologic augmentation for rotator cuff repair. Annals of the New York Academy of Sciences. 2016;**1383**(1):97-114

[23] Pauly S, Klatte F, Strobel C, Schmidmaier G, Greiner S, Scheibel M, et al. BMP-2 and BMP-7 affect human rotator cuff tendon cells in vitro. Journal of Shoulder and Elbow Surgery. 2012;**21**(4):464-473

[24] Zhou Q, Zhang J-H, Yuan S, Shao J-H, Cai Z-Y, Chen S, et al. A new insight of Kartogenin induced the mesenchymal stem cells (MSCs) selectively differentiate into chondrocytes by activating the bone morphogenetic protein 7 (BMP-7)/Smad5 pathway. Medical Science Monitor. 2019;**25**:4960-4967

[25] Lee K-W, Lee J-S, Kim Y-S, Shim Y-B, Jang J-W, Lee K-I. Effective healing of chronic rotator cuff injury using recombinant bone morphogenetic protein-2 coated dermal patch in vivo. Journal of Biomedical Materials Research. Part B, Applied Biomaterials. 2017;**105**(7):1840-1846

[26] Kabuto Y, Morihara T, Sukenari T, Kida Y, Oda R, Arai Y, et al. Stimulation of rotator cuff repair by sustained release of bone morphogenetic Protein-7 using a Gelatin hydrogel sheet. Tissue Engineering. Part A. 2015;**21**(13-14):2025-2033

[27] Longo UG, Lamberti A, Maffulli N, Denaro V. Tissue engineered biological augmentation for tendon healing: A systematic review. British Medical Bulletin. 2011;**98**:31-59

[28] Seeherman HJ, Archambault JM, Rodeo SA, Simon Turner A, Zekas L,

D'Augusta D, et al. rhBMP-12 accelerates healing of rotator cuff repairs in a sheep model. The Journal of Bone and Joint Surgery-American Volume. 2008;**90**:2206-2219. DOI: 10.2106/jbjs.g.00742

[29] Lamplot JD, Angeline M, Angeles J, Beederman M, Wagner E, Rastegar F, et al. Distinct effects of platelet-rich plasma and BMP13 on rotator cuff tendon injury healing in a rat model. The American Journal of Sports Medicine. 2014;**42**(12):2877-2887

[30] Greiner S, Ide J, Van Noort A, Mochizuki Y, Ochi H, Marraffino S, et al. Local rhBMP-12 on an absorbable collagen sponge as an adjuvant therapy for rotator cuff repair—A Phase 1, randomized, standard of care control, multicenter study. The American Journal of Sports Medicine. 2015;**43**:1994-2004. DOI: 10.1177/0363546515584756

[31] Isaac C, Gharaibeh B, Witt M, Wright VJ, Huard J. Biologic approaches to enhance rotator cuff healing after injury. Journal of Shoulder and Elbow Surgery. 2012;**21**(2):181-190

[32] Uggen C, Dines J, McGarry M, Grande D, Lee T, Limpisvasti O. The effect of recombinant human platelet-derived growth factor BB–coated sutures on rotator cuff healing in a sheep model. Arthroscopy: The Journal of Arthroscopic & Related Surgery. 2010;**26**:1456-1462. DOI: 10.1016/j.arthro.2010.02.025

[33] Chan BP, Fu SC, Qin L, Rolf C, Chan KM. Supplementation-time dependence of growth factors in promoting tendon healing. Clinical Orthopaedics and Related Research. 2006;**448**:240-247

[34] Gulotta LV, Rodeo SA. Growth factors for rotator cuff repair. Clinics in Sports Medicine. 2009;**28**(1):13-23

[35] Tokunaga T, Ide J, Arimura H, Nakamura T, Uehara Y, Sakamoto H, et al. Local application of gelatin hydrogel sheets impregnated with platelet-derived growth factor BB promotes tendon-to-bone healing after rotator cuff repair in rats. Arthroscopy. 2015;**31**(8):1482-1491

[36] Kovacevic D, Gulotta LV, Ying L, Ehteshami JR, Deng X-H, Rodeo SA. rhPDGF-BB promotes early healing in a rat rotator cuff repair model. Clinical Orthopaedics & Related Research. 2015;**473**:1644-1654. DOI: 10.1007/s11999-014-4020-0

[37] Molloy T, Wang Y, Murrell G. The roles of growth factors in tendon and ligament healing. Sports Medicine. 2003;**33**(5):381-394

[38] Manning CN, Mike Kim H, Sakiyama-Elbert S, Galatz LM, Havlioglu N, Thomopoulos S. Sustained delivery of transforming growth factor beta three enhances tendon-to-bone healing in a rat model. Journal of Orthopaedic Research. 2011;**29**:1099-1105. DOI: 10.1002/jor.21301

[39] Kim HM, Galatz LM, Das R, Havlioglu N, Rothermich SY, Thomopoulos S. The role of transforming growth factor beta isoforms in tendon-to-bone healing. Connective Tissue Research. 2011;**52**(2):87-98

[40] Yoon JP, Lee C-H, Jung JW, Lee H-J, Lee Y-S, Kim J-Y, et al. Sustained delivery of transforming growth factor β1 by use of absorbable alginate scaffold enhances rotator cuff healing in a rabbit model. The American Journal of Sports Medicine. 2018;**46**:1441-1450. DOI: 10.1177/0363546518757759

[41] Yoon JP, Kim H-M, Choi J-H, Kang HR, Kim DH, Choi YS, et al. Effect of a porous suture containing

transforming growth factor beta 1 on healing after rotator cuff repair in a rat model. The American Journal of Sports Medicine. 2021;**49**:3050-3058. DOI: 10.1177/03635465211028547

[42] Takahashi S, Nakajima M, Kobayashi M, Wakabayashi I, Miyakoshi N, Minagawa H, et al. Effect of recombinant basic fibroblast growth factor (bFGF) on fibroblast-like cells from human rotator cuff tendon. The Tohoku Journal of Experimental Medicine. 2002;**198**(4):207-214

[43] Ide J, Kikukawa K, Hirose J, Iyama K-I, Sakamoto H, Fujimoto T, et al. The effect of a local application of fibroblast growth factor-2 on tendon-to-bone remodeling in rats with acute injury and repair of the supraspinatus tendon. Journal of Shoulder and Elbow Surgery. 2009;**18**(3):391-398

[44] Lu Y, Lee JS, Nemke B, Baer G, Graf BK, Murphy WL, et al. Histologic evaluation of suture material loaded with basic fibroblast growth factor (bFGF) on acute rotator cuff repair in an ovine model. Current Orthopaedic Practice. 2011;**22**:425-431. DOI: 10.1097/bco.0b013e3182282cd7

[45] Peterson DR, Ohashi KL, Aberman HM, Piza PA, Crockett HC, Fernandez JI, et al. Evaluation of a collagen-coated, resorbable fiber scaffold loaded with a peptide basic fibroblast growth factor mimetic in a sheep model of rotator cuff repair. Journal of Shoulder and Elbow Surgery. 2015;**24**:1764-1773. DOI: 10.1016/j.jse.2015.06.009

[46] Tokunaga T, Karasugi T, Arimura H, Yonemitsu R, Sakamoto H, Ide J, et al. Enhancement of rotator cuff tendon–bone healing with fibroblast growth factor 2 impregnated in gelatin hydrogel sheets in a rabbit model. Journal of Shoulder and Elbow Surgery. 2017;**26**:1708-1717. DOI: 10.1016/j.jse.2017.03.020

[47] Yonemitsu R, Tokunaga T, Shukunami C, Ideo K, Arimura H, Karasugi T, et al. Fibroblast growth factor 2 enhances tendon-to-bone healing in a rat rotator cuff repair of chronic tears. The American Journal of Sports Medicine. 2019;**47**:1701-1712. DOI: 10.1177/0363546519836959

[48] Kataoka T, Mifune Y, Inui A, Nishimoto H, Kurosawa T, Yamaura K, et al. Combined therapy of platelet-rich plasma and basic fibroblast growth factor using gelatin-hydrogel sheet for rotator cuff healing in rat models. Journal of Orthopaedic Surgery and Research. 2021;**16**(1):605

[49] Chahal J, Van Thiel GS, Mall N, Heard W, Bach BR, Cole BJ, et al. The role of platelet-rich plasma in arthroscopic rotator cuff repair: A systematic review with quantitative synthesis. Arthroscopy. 2012;**28**(11):1718-1727

[50] Jo CH, Kim JE, Yoon KS, Lee JH, Kang SB, Lee JH, et al. Does platelet-rich plasma accelerate recovery after rotator cuff repair? A prospective cohort study. The American Journal of Sports Medicine. 2011;**39**:2082-2090. DOI: 10.1177/0363546511413454

[51] Zhang C, Wu J, Li X, Wang Z, Lu WW, Wong T-M. Current biological strategies to enhance surgical treatment for rotator cuff repair. Frontiers in Bioengineering and Biotechnology. 2021;**9**:657584

[52] Ersen A, Demirhan M, Atalar AC, Kapicioğlu M, Baysal G. Platelet-rich plasma for enhancing surgical rotator cuff repair: Evaluation and comparison of two application methods in a rat model. Archives of Orthopaedic and Trauma Surgery. 2014;**134**(3):405-411

[53] Dohan Ehrenfest DM, Rasmusson L, Albrektsson T. Classification of platelet concentrates: From pure platelet-rich plasma (P-PRP) to leucocyte- and platelet-rich fibrin (L-PRF). Trends in Biotechnology. 2009;**27**(3):158-167

[54] Otarodifard K, Bruce Canham R, Galatz LM. Biologic augmentation of rotator cuff repair. Seminars in Arthroplasty. 2014;**25**:220-225. DOI: 10.1053/j.sart.2015.04.009

[55] Anitua E, Cugat R, Sánchez M. Platelet Rich Plasma in Orthopaedics and Sports Medicine. Cham, Switzerland: Springer; 2018. p. 276

[56] Kobayashi Y, Saita Y, Nishio H, Ikeda H, Takazawa Y, Nagao M, et al. Leukocyte concentration and composition in platelet-rich plasma (PRP) influences the growth factor and protease concentrations. Journal of Orthopaedic Science. 2016;**21**:683-689. DOI: 10.1016/j.jos.2016.07.009

[57] Kim SJ, Kim EK, Kim SJ, Song DH. Effects of bone marrow aspirate concentrate and platelet-rich plasma on patients with partial tear of the rotator cuff tendon. Journal of Orthopaedic Surgery and Research. 2018;**13**:1-7. DOI: 10.1186/s13018-017-0693-x

[58] Ebert JR, Wang A, Smith A, Nairn R, Breidahl W, Zheng MH, et al. A midterm evaluation of postoperative platelet-rich plasma injections on arthroscopic supraspinatus repair: A randomized controlled trial. The American Journal of Sports Medicine. 2017;**45**:2965-2974. DOI: 10.1177/0363546517719048

[59] Andia I, Martin JI, Maffulli N. Advances with platelet rich plasma therapies for tendon regeneration. Expert Opinion on Biological Therapy. 2018;**18**:389-398. DOI: 10.1080/14712598.2018.1424626

[60] Lu HH, Vo JM, Chin HS, Lin J, Cozin M, Tsay R, et al. Controlled delivery of platelet-rich plasma-derived growth factors for bone formation. Journal of Biomedical Materials Research Part A. 2008;**86A**:1128-1136. DOI: 10.1002/jbm.a.31740

[61] Carr JB, Rodeo SA. Rotator cuff repair: A biological approach to improve outcomes. Operative Techniques in Sports Medicine. 2020;**28**:150757. DOI: 10.1016/j.otsm.2020.150757

[62] Zhou Y, Wang JH-C. PRP treatment efficacy for tendinopathy: A review of basic science studies. BioMed Research International. 2016;**2016**:1-8. DOI: 10.1155/2016/9103792

[63] Zhang J, Wang JH-C. Platelet-rich plasma releasate promotes differentiation of tendon stem cells into active tenocytes. The American Journal of Sports Medicine. 2010;**38**(12):2477-2486

[64] Anitua E, Andí I, Sanchez M, Azofra J, del Mar Zalduendo M, de la Fuente M, et al. Autologous preparations rich in growth factors promote proliferation and induce VEGF and HGF production by human tendon cells in culture. Journal of Orthopaedic Research. 2005;**23**:281-286. DOI: 10.1016/j.orthres.2004.08.015

[65] Hoppe S, Alini M, Benneker LM, Milz S, Boileau P, Zumstein MA. Tenocytes of chronic rotator cuff tendon tears can be stimulated by platelet-released growth factors. Journal of Shoulder and Elbow Surgery. 2013;**22**(3):340-349

[66] Dolkart O, Chechik O, Zarfati Y, Brosh T, Alhajajra F, Maman E. A single dose of platelet-rich plasma improves the organization and strength of a surgically repaired rotator cuff tendon in rats. Archives of Orthopaedic and Trauma Surgery. 2014;**134**(9):1271-1277

[67] Kesikburun S, Tan AK, Yılmaz B, Yaşar E, Yazıcıoğlu K. Platelet-rich plasma injections in the treatment of chronic rotator cuff tendinopathy. The American Journal of Sports Medicine. 2013;**41**:2609-2616. DOI: 10.1177/0363546513496542

[68] Shams A, El-Sayed M, Gamal O, Ewes W. Subacromial injection of autologous platelet-rich plasma versus corticosteroid for the treatment of symptomatic partial rotator cuff tears. European Journal of Orthopaedic Surgery and Traumatology. 2016;**26**(8):837-842

[69] Jo CH, Shin JS, Lee YG, Shin WH, Kim H, Lee SY, et al. Platelet-rich plasma for arthroscopic repair of large to massive rotator cuff tears: A randomized, single-blind, parallel-group trial. The American Journal of Sports Medicine. 2013;**41**(10):2240-2248

[70] Hurley ET, Lim Fat D, Moran CJ, Mullett H. The efficacy of platelet-rich plasma and platelet-rich fibrin in arthroscopic rotator cuff repair: A meta-analysis of randomized controlled trials. The American Journal of Sports Medicine. 2019;**47**(3):753-761

[71] Cavendish PA, Everhart JS, DiBartola AC, Eikenberry AD, Cvetanovich GL, Flanigan DC. The effect of perioperative platelet-rich plasma injections on postoperative failure rates following rotator cuff repair: A systematic review with meta-analysis. Journal of Shoulder and Elbow Surgery. 2020;**29**(5):1059-1070

[72] Pandey V, Bandi A, Madi S, Agarwal L, Acharya KKV, Maddukuri S, et al. Does application of moderately concentrated platelet-rich plasma improve clinical and structural outcome after arthroscopic repair of medium-sized to large rotator cuff tear? A randomized controlled trial. Journal of Shoulder and Elbow Surgery. 2016;**25**(8):1312-1322

[73] Jo CH, Shin JS, Shin WH, Lee SY, Yoon KS, Shin S. Platelet-rich plasma for arthroscopic repair of medium to large rotator cuff tears: A randomized controlled trial. The American Journal of Sports Medicine. 2015;**43**(9):2102-2110

[74] Randelli P, Arrigoni P, Ragone V, Aliprandi A, Cabitza P. Platelet rich plasma in arthroscopic rotator cuff repair: A prospective RCT study, 2-year follow-up. Journal of Shoulder and Elbow Surgery. 2011;**20**(4):518-528

[75] Malavolta EA, Gracitelli MEC, Assunção JH, Ferreira Neto AA, Bordalo-Rodrigues M, de Camargo OP. Clinical and structural evaluations of rotator cuff repair with and without added platelet-rich plasma at 5-year follow-up: A prospective randomized study. The American Journal of Sports Medicine. 2018;**46**(13):3134-3141

[76] Zhao J-G, Zhao L, Jiang Y-X, Wang Z-L, Wang J, Zhang P. Platelet-rich plasma in arthroscopic rotator cuff repair: A meta-analysis of randomized controlled trials. Arthroscopy: The Journal of Arthroscopic & Related Surgery. 2015;**31**:125-135. DOI: 10.1016/j.arthro.2014.08.008

[77] Charousset C, Zaoui A, Bellaïche L, Piterman M. Does autologous leukocyte-platelet-rich plasma improve tendon healing in arthroscopic repair of large or massive rotator cuff tears? Arthroscopy. 2014;**30**(4):428-435

[78] Rodeo SA, Delos D, Williams RJ, Adler RS, Pearle A, Warren RF. The effect of platelet-rich fibrin matrix on rotator cuff tendon healing: A prospective, randomized clinical study. The

American Journal of Sports Medicine. 2012;**40**(6):1234-1241

[79] Ruiz-Moneo P, Molano-Muñoz J, Prieto E, Algorta J. Plasma rich in growth factors in arthroscopic rotator cuff repair: A randomized, double-blind, controlled clinical trial. Arthroscopy. 2013;**29**(1):2-9

[80] Randelli PS, Stoppani CA, Santarsiero G, Nocerino E, Menon A. Platelet rich plasma in arthroscopic rotator cuff repair: Clinical and radiological results of a prospective RCT study at 10-year follow-up. Arthroscopy. 2021;**38**(1)51-61. DOI: 10.1016/j.arthro.2021.05.017

[81] Gulotta LV, Kovacevic D, Ehteshami JR, Dagher E, Packer JD, Rodeo SA. Application of bone marrow-derived mesenchymal stem cells in a rotator cuff repair model. The American Journal of Sports Medicine. 2009;**37**:2126-2133. DOI: 10.1177/0363546509339582

[82] Gulotta LV, Kovacevic D, Packer JD, Deng XH, Rodeo SA. Bone marrow–derived mesenchymal stem cells transduced with scleraxis improve rotator cuff healing in a rat model. The American Journal of Sports Medicine. 2011;**39**:1282-1289. DOI: 10.1177/0363546510395485

[83] Yokoya S, Mochizuki Y, Natsu K, Omae H, Nagata Y, Ochi M. Rotator cuff regeneration using a bioabsorbable material with bone marrow–derived mesenchymal stem cells in a rabbit model. The American Journal of Sports Medicine. 2012;**40**:1259-1268. DOI: 10.1177/0363546512442343

[84] Hernigou P, Flouzat Lachaniette CH, Delambre J, Zilber S, Duffiet P, Chevallier N, et al. Biologic augmentation of rotator cuff repair with mesenchymal stem cells during arthroscopy improves healing and prevents further tears: A case-controlled study. International Orthopaedics. 2014;**38**(9):1811-1818

[85] Degen RM, Carbone A, Carballo C, Zong J, Chen T, Lebaschi A, et al. The effect of purified human bone marrow–derived mesenchymal stem cells on rotator cuff tendon healing in an athymic rat. Arthroscopy: The Journal of Arthroscopic & Related Surgery. 2016;**32**:2435-2443. DOI: 10.1016/j.arthro.2016.04.019

[86] Thangarajah T, Sanghani-Kerai A, Henshaw F, Lambert SM, Pendegrass CJ, Blunn GW. Application of a demineralized cortical bone matrix and bone marrow–derived mesenchymal stem cells in a model of chronic rotator cuff degeneration. The American Journal of Sports Medicine. 2018;**46**:98-108. DOI: 10.1177/0363546517727512

[87] Han L, Fang W-L, Jin B, Xu S-C, Zheng X, Hu Y-G. Enhancement of tendon-bone healing after rotator cuff injuries using combined therapy with mesenchymal stem cells and platelet rich plasma. European Review for Medical and Pharmacological Sciences. 2019;**23**(20):9075-9084

[88] Oh JH, Chung SW, Kim SH, Chung JY, Kim JY. 2013 Neer Award: Effect of the adipose-derived stem cell for the improvement of fatty degeneration and rotator cuff healing in rabbit model. Journal of Shoulder and Elbow Surgery. 2014;**23**(4):445-455

[89] Mora MV, Antuña SA, Arranz MG, Carrascal MT, Barco R. Application of adipose tissue-derived stem cells in a rat rotator cuff repair model. Injury. 2014;**45**:S22-S27. DOI: 10.1016/s0020-1383(14)70006-3

[90] Lipner J, Shen H, Cavinatto L, Liu W, Havlioglu N, Xia Y, et al. In vivo evaluation of adipose-derived stromal cells delivered with a nanofiber scaffold for tendon-to-bone repair. Tissue Engineering. Part A. 2015;**21**(21-22):2766-2774

[91] Chen H-S, Su Y-T, Chan T-M, Su Y-J, Syu W-S, Harn H-J, et al. Human adipose-derived stem cells accelerate the restoration of tensile strength of tendon and alleviate the progression of rotator cuff injury in a rat model. Cell Transplantation. 2015;**24**:509-520. DOI: 10.3727/096368915x686968

[92] Rothrauff BB, Smith CA, Ferrer GA, Novaretti JV, Pauyo T, Chao T, et al. The effect of adipose-derived stem cells on enthesis healing after repair of acute and chronic massive rotator cuff tears in rats. Journal of Shoulder and Elbow Surgery. 2019;**28**(4):654-664

[93] Wang C, Song W, Chen B, Liu X, He Y. Exosomes isolated from adipose-derived stem cells: A new cell-free approach to prevent the muscle degeneration associated with torn rotator cuffs. The American Journal of Sports Medicine. 2019;**47**(13):3247-3255

[94] Park G-Y, Kwon DR, Lee SC. Regeneration of full-thickness rotator cuff tendon tear after ultrasound-guided injection with umbilical cord blood-derived mesenchymal stem cells in a rabbit model. Stem Cells Translational Medicine. 2015;**4**:1344-1351. DOI: 10.5966/sctm.2015-0040

[95] Kwon DR, Park G-Y, Lee SC. Treatment of full-thickness rotator cuff tendon tear using umbilical cord blood-derived mesenchymal stem cells and Polydeoxyribonucleotides in a rabbit model. Stem Cells International. 2018;(1):1-11. DOI: 10.1155/2018/7146384

[96] Kwon DR, Park G-Y, Moon YS, Lee SC. Therapeutic effects of umbilical cord blood-derived mesenchymal stem cells combined with polydeoxyribonucleotides on full-thickness rotator cuff tendon tear in a rabbit model. Cell Transplantation. 2018;**27**:1613-1622. DOI: 10.1177/0963689718799040

[97] Kwon DR, Jung S, Jang J, Park G-Y, Moon YS, Lee SC. A 3-dimensional bioprinted scaffold with human umbilical cord blood–mesenchymal stem cells improves regeneration of chronic full-thickness rotator cuff tear in a rabbit model. The American Journal of Sports Medicine. 2020;**48**:947-958. DOI: 10.1177/0363546520904022

[98] Mocini F, Monteleone AS, Piazza P, Cardona V, Vismara V, Messinese P, et al. The role of adipose derived stem cells in the treatment of rotator cuff tears: From basic science to clinical application. Orthopaedic Review. 2020;**12**(Suppl 1):8682

[99] Zuk PA, Zhu M, Mizuno H, Huang J, Futrell JW, Katz AJ, et al. Multilineage cells from human adipose tissue: Implications for cell-based therapies. Tissue Engineering. 2001;**7**(2):211-228

[100] Kim YS, Sung CH, Chung SH, Kwak SJ, Koh YG. Does an injection of adipose-derived mesenchymal stem cells loaded in fibrin glue influence rotator cuff repair outcomes? A clinical and magnetic resonance imaging study. The American Journal of Sports Medicine. 2017;**45**(9):2010-2018

[101] Jo CH, Chai JW, Jeong EC, Oh S, Kim PS, Yoon JY, et al. Intratendinous injection of autologous adipose tissue-derived mesenchymal stem cells for the treatment of rotator cuff disease: A first-in-human trial. Stem Cells. 2018;**36**(9):1441-1450

[102] Jo CH, Chai JW, Jeong EC, Oh S, Yoon KS. Intratendinous injection of mesenchymal stem cells for the treatment of rotator cuff disease: A 2-year follow-up study. Arthroscopy. 2020;**36**(4):971-980

[103] Lhee S-H, Jo YH, Kim BY, Nam BM, Nemeno JG, Lee S, et al. Novel supplier of mesenchymal stem cell: Subacromial bursa. Transplantation Proceedings. 2013;**45**(8):3118-3121

[104] Morikawa D, Muench LN, Baldino JB, Kia C, Johnson J, Otto A, et al. Comparison of preparation techniques for isolating subacromial bursa-derived cells as a potential augment for rotator cuff repair. Arthroscopy. 2020;**36**(1):80-85

[105] Morikawa D, Johnson JD, Kia C, McCarthy MBR, Macken C, Bellas N, et al. Examining the potency of subacromial bursal cells as a potential augmentation for rotator cuff healing: An in vitro study. Arthroscopy: The Journal of Arthroscopic & Related Surgery. 2019;**35**:2978-2988. DOI: 10.1016/j.arthro.2019.05.024

[106] Muench LN, Baldino JB, Berthold DP, Kia C, Lebaschi A, Cote MP, et al. Subacromial bursa-derived cells demonstrate high proliferation potential regardless of patient demographics and rotator cuff tear characteristics. Arthroscopy. 2020;**36**(11):2794-2802

[107] Landry A, Levy BJ, McCarthy MB, Muench LN, Uyeki C, Berthold DP, et al. Analysis of time to form colony units for connective tissue progenitor cells (stem cells) harvested from concentrated bone marrow aspirate and subacromial Bursa tissue in patients undergoing rotator cuff repair. Sports Medicine, Arthroscopy, Rehabilitation, Therapy & Technology: SMARTT. 2020;**2**(5):e629-e636

[108] Freislederer F, Dittrich M, Scheibel M. Biological augmentation with subacromial bursa in arthroscopic rotator cuff repair. Arthroscopy Techniques. 2019;**8**(7):e741-e747

[109] Yates EW, Rupani A, Foley GT, Khan WS, Cartmell S, Anand SJ. Ligament tissue engineering and its potential role in anterior cruciate ligament reconstruction. Stem Cells International. 2012;**2012**:438125

[110] Mozafari M, Rajadas J, Kaplan D. Nanoengineered biomaterials for regenerative medicine. Cambridge, MA: Elsevier; 2018. p. 516

[111] Chen J, Xu J, Wang A, Zheng M. Scaffolds for tendon and ligament repair: Review of the efficacy of commercial products. Expert Review of Medical Devices. 2009;**6**(1):61-73

[112] Fan H, Liu H, Toh SL, Goh JCH. Anterior cruciate ligament regeneration using mesenchymal stem cells and silk scaffold in large animal model. Biomaterials. 2009;**30**:4967-4977. DOI: 10.1016/j.biomaterials.2009.05.048

[113] Teh TKH, Toh S-L, Goh JCH. Aligned hybrid silk scaffold for enhanced differentiation of mesenchymal stem cells into ligament fibroblasts. Tissue Engineering. Part C, Methods. 2011;**17**(6):687-703

[114] Thaker H, Sharma AK. Engaging stem cells for customized tendon regeneration. Stem Cells International. 2012;**2012**:309187

[115] Gross G, Hoffmann A. Therapeutic strategies for tendon healing based on novel biomaterials, factors and cells. Pathobiology. 2013;**80**(4):203-210

[116] Thon S, Savoie FH 3rd. Rotator cuff repair: Patch the shoulder. Arthroscopy. 2019;**35**(4):1014-1015

[117] Voss A, McCarthy MB, Hoberman A, Cote MP, Imhoff AB, Mazzocca AD, et al. Extracellular matrix of current biological scaffolds promotes the differentiation potential of mesenchymal stem cells. Arthroscopy: The Journal of Arthroscopic & Related Surgery. 2016;**32**:2381-92.e1. DOI: 10.1016/j.arthro.2016.04.033

[118] Bokor DJ, Sonnabend D, Deady L, Cass B, Young A, Van Kampen C, et al. Evidence of healing of partial-thickness rotator cuff tears following arthroscopic augmentation with a collagen implant: A 2-year MRI follow-up. Muscle, Ligaments and Tendons Journal. 2016;**6**(1):16-25

[119] Zhang X, Bogdanowicz D, Erisken C, Lee NM, Lu HH. Biomimetic scaffold design for functional and integrative tendon repair. Journal of Shoulder and Elbow Surgery. 2012;**21**(2):266-277

[120] Ricchetti ET, Aurora A, Iannotti JP, Derwin KA. Scaffold devices for rotator cuff repair. Journal of Shoulder and Elbow Surgery. 2012;**21**(2):251-265

[121] Yeganegi M, Kandel RA, Santerre JP. Characterization of a biodegradable electrospun polyurethane nanofiber scaffold: Mechanical properties and cytotoxicity. Acta Biomaterialia. 2010;**6**(10):3847-3855

[122] Moffat KL, Kwei AS-P, Spalazzi JP, Doty SB, Levine WN, Lu HH. Novel nanofiber-based scaffold for rotator cuff repair and augmentation. Tissue Engineering. Part A. 2009;**15**(1):115-126

[123] Sahoo S, Ouyang H, Goh JC-H, Tay TE, Toh SL. Characterization of a novel polymeric scaffold for potential application in tendon/ligament tissue engineering. Tissue Engineering. 2006;**12**(1):91-99

[124] Taylor ED, Nair LS, Nukavarapu SP, McLaughlin S, Laurencin CT. Novel nanostructured scaffolds as therapeutic replacement options for rotator cuff disease. The Journal of Bone and Joint Surgery. American Volume. 2010;**92**(Suppl 2):170-179

[125] Cross LM, Thakur A, Jalili NA, Detamore M, Gaharwar AK. Nanoengineered biomaterials for repair and regeneration of orthopedic tissue interfaces. Acta Biomaterialia. 2016;**42**:2-17

[126] Liu W, Lipner J, Xie J, Manning CN, Thomopoulos S, Xia Y. Nanofiber scaffolds with gradients in mineral content for spatial control of osteogenesis. ACS Applied Materials & Interfaces. 2014;**6**(4):2842-2849

[127] Nuss CA, Huegel J, Boorman-Padgett JF, Choi DS, Weiss SN, Vournakis J, et al. Poly-N-acetyl glucosamine (sNAG) enhances early rotator cuff tendon healing in a rat model. Annals of Biomedical Engineering. 2017;**45**(12):2826-2836

[128] Chen C-H, Chang C-H, Wang K-C, Su C-I, Liu H-T, Yu C-M, et al. Enhancement of rotator cuff tendon–bone healing with injectable periosteum progenitor cells-BMP-2 hydrogel in vivo. Knee Surgery, Sports Traumatology, Arthroscopy. 2011;**19**:1597-1607. DOI: 10.1007/s00167-010-1373-0

[129] Buchmann S, Sandmann GH, Walz L, Reichel T, Beitzel K, Wexel G, et al. Growth factor release by vesicular phospholipid gels: In-vitro results and application for rotator cuff repair in a rat model. BMC Musculoskeletal Disorders. 2015;**16**:82

[130] Tian W, Schulze S, Brandl M, Winter G. Vesicular phospholipid gel-based depot formulations for

pharmaceutical proteins: Development and in vitro evaluation. Journal of Controlled Release. 2010;**142**(3):319-325

[131] Del Buono A, Oliva F, Longo UG, Rodeo SA, Orchard J, Denaro V, et al. Metalloproteases and rotator cuff disease. Journal of Shoulder and Elbow Surgery. 2012;**21**(2):200-208

[132] Lo IKY, Marchuk LL, Hollinshead R, Hart DA, Frank CB. Matrix metalloproteinase and tissue inhibitor of matrix metalloproteinase mRNA levels are specifically altered in torn rotator cuff tendons. The American Journal of Sports Medicine. 2004;**32**(5):1223-1229

[133] Bedi A, Fox AJS, Kovacevic D, Deng X-H, Warren RF, Rodeo SA. Doxycycline-mediated inhibition of matrix metalloproteinases improves healing after rotator cuff repair. The American Journal of Sports Medicine. 2010;**38**(2):308-317

[134] Bedi A, Kovacevic D, Hettrich C, Gulotta LV, Ehteshami JR, Warren RF, et al. The effect of matrix metalloproteinase inhibition on tendon-to-bone healing in a rotator cuff repair model. Journal of Shoulder and Elbow Surgery. 2010;**19**:384-391. DOI: 10.1016/j.jse.2009.07.010

[135] Eliasberg CD, Dar A, Jensen AR, Murray IR, Hardy WR, Kowalski TJ, et al. Perivascular stem cells diminish muscle atrophy following massive rotator cuff tears in a small animal model. The Journal of Bone and Joint Surgery. American Volume. 2017;**99**(4):331-341

[136] Dyrna F, Zakko P, Pauzenberger L, McCarthy MB, Mazzocca AD, Dyment NA. Human subacromial bursal cells display superior engraftment versus bone marrow stromal cells in murine tendon repair. The American Journal of Sports Medicine. 2018;**46**:3511-3520. DOI: 10.1177/0363546518802842

[137] Novak ML, Koh TJ. Macrophage phenotypes during tissue repair. Journal of Leukocyte Biology. 2013;**93**:875-881. DOI: 10.1189/jlb.1012512

[138] Chamberlain CS, Clements AEB, Kink JA, Choi U, Baer GS, Halanski MA, et al. Extracellular vesicle-educated macrophages promote early achilles tendon healing. Stem cells. 2019;**37**:652-662. DOI: 10.1002/stem.2988

[139] Dines JS, Grande DA, ElAttrache N, Dines DM. Biologics in shoulder surgery: Suture augmentation and coating to enhance tendon repair. Techniques in Orthopaedics. 2007;**22**:20-25. DOI: 10.1097/01.bto.0000261867.07628.80

[140] Lee N, Robinson J, Lu H. Biomimetic strategies for engineering composite tissues. Current Opinion in Biotechnology. 2016;**40**:64-74

[141] Washington KS, Shemshaki NS, Laurencin CT. The role of nanomaterials and biological agents on rotator cuff regeneration. Regenerative Engineering and Translational Medicine. 2020;**7**:440-449. DOI: 10.1007/s40883-020-00171-1

Chapter 2

Single-Row Rotator Cuff Repair

Amhaz Escanlar S., Jorge Mora A. and Pino Miguez J.

Abstract

Rotator cuff tears are a common cause of pain and disability among adults. Partial tears are usually treated conservatively. Complete tears might be treated conservatively in some cases; however, surgical repair is often performed in selected cases and situations where conservative treatment fails to restore function and pain relief. In addition, some patients with acute tears might be good candidates for acute surgical repair, as will be studied in this chapter. A plethora of techniques is available to repair rotator cuff tears. Among these, the surgeon faces the dilemma to choose the best treatment for the patient. Open techniques were the gold standard in the 1990s. However, the advent of arthroscopy has led the shoulder and sports surgeon community towards these. Arthroscopic rotator cuff repair has become the gold standard nowadays despite the lack of proper evidence to support this change. Furthermore, simple single-row repairs had been discarded favouring double-row techniques, yet new evidence supports the use of the former due to similar results, simplicity and cost-effectiveness. This chapter examines current evidence to help the surgeon decide between open and minimally invasive techniques and select suitable repair configurations.

Keywords: rotator, cuff, single-row, transosseous, double-row, mini-open, arthroscopy

1. Introduction

Rotator cuff tears are commonly seen in the orthopedic surgeon clinic, even more in the shoulder and elbow subspecialized professional practice. Different muscles form the rotator cuff: subscapularis, supraspinatus, infraspinatus, teres minor, and some authors also include the teres major due to its role as an internal rotator. The primary role of the rotator cuff is to stabilize the humeral head regarding the glenoid to allow the deltoid to perform the elevation of the arm. In addition, the rotator cuff externally rotates the glenohumeral joint (infraspinatus and teres minor) and contributes to internal rotation (subscapularis, assisted by the pectoralis major, teres major and latissimus dorsi) [1].

Patients with rotator cuff tears mainly complain of pain during daily living activities but also at night, when the pain can likewise interfere with proper resting. Moreover, a significant tear may impair function, limiting the active range of motion and can be the culprit of premature glenohumeral arthritis. Loss of external rotation, sometimes isolated, may appear in the onset of a posterior rotator cuff tear [1, 2].

Rotator cuff tears are expected after 60 years old. They correspond with the Neer type 3 stage and can be identified in about 20–30% of the patients in this age group. Beyond 80 years old, the ratio of patients suffering from cuff tears rises to more than 60%. However, the symptoms do not correlate with the presence of tears or even the size or retraction. Most patients do not seek advice from an orthopedic surgeon and do not demand a surgical intervention. More than half of the patients where a tear is identified will also suffer from a tear in their contralateral shoulder, especially in those older than 60 years [2–7].

1.1 Risk factors

Several risk factors have been identified concerning cuff tears. Age, as it was aforementioned, is the most significant. However, others such as smoking, hypercholesterolemia, diabetes, hypo or hyperthyroidism, trauma, scapular dyskinesia and kyphosis also play a critical role in the development and progression of cuff tears [7–15].

1.2 Classification

A plethora of classifications for rotator cuff tears has been described since the pathology became more interesting for the orthopedic community.

Neer described the evolution of rotator cuff disease in three stages. First, in individuals younger than 40 years, one can observe oedema and hemorrhage in the rotator cuff. In a second stage, the disease evolves in individuals between 40 and 60 years old, and fibrotic and tendinosis phenomena might be observed. Finally, in a third stage, usually, in patients older than 60 years, a tendon rupture is observed. Probably a fourth stage would involve rotator cuff arthropathy, with cephalad migration of the humeral head and degenerative osteoarthritis at the level of the glenoid as well as in the humeral head [15, 16].

Some authors have advocated for a classification based on tear size. Cofield in 1982 described four types of tears: small (<1 cm) medium (1–3 cm) large (3–5 cm) massive (>5 cm) [17].

Bateman also described a four-group classification based on the size: Grade 1 (<1 cm after debridement), Grade 2 (1–3 cm, after debridement), Grade 3 (<5 cm) and Grade 4 (global tear with no cuff left) [18].

Harryman described a classification based on the number of injured tendons. It is commonly accepted in Europe that a complete tear of two or more tendons should be considered massive, and concerns about reparability should arise [19].

Ellman and Gartsman introduced in 1993 a classification differentiating partial-thickness and full-thickness tears. Partial tears were classified in grade 1 (<3 mm deep, <25% thickness), grade 2 (3–6 mm, <50%) and grade 3 (>6 mm, >50%). The partial tear classification system is accepted worldwide as it helps in treatment selection, as discussed in the next section. These authors also proposed a full-thickness classification based on tear-shaped, which has been judged useful and is currently used worldwide. Five groups were described: crescent shape, L shape, Reverse L, trapezoidal shape and massive tears [20, 21].

Concerning partial tears, Snyder clarified that a distinction between articular and bursal tears is mandatory as the criteria for surgery are different.

Fox and Romeo described a specific classification for subscapularis tears in 2003. Four types were proposed: Type 1, partial thickness; Type 2, complete tear of the upper 25%; Type 3, a complete tear of the upper 50%; Type 4, complete rupture of the subscapularis tendon [22].

Other authors prefer to classify tears about the retraction, as it can help the surgeon assess reparability before the operation. Patte described in 1990 three groups: Stage 1, where the tendon stump is adjacent to its insertion; Stage 2, with a tendon stump at the level of the humeral head; Stage 3, where the tendon is at the glenoid level or even more medial.

Patte also described a classification in the sagittal plane based on six segments: Segment 1, isolated subscapularis tear; Segment 2, isolated rotator interval tear; Segment 3, isolated supraspinatus tear; Segment 4, supraspinatus and upper one-half of the infraspinatus; Segment 5, complete supraspinatus and infraspinatus; and Segment 6, complete cuff rupture [23].

Finally, some authors prefer a classification based on tissue quality and atrophy. Currently, the classification proposed by Goutallier in 1994 is the most accepted and used. The author described stage 0, corresponding with a normal muscle. Stage 1, some fatty streaks; Stage 2, less than 50% of fatty atrophy; Stage 3, more than 50% of fat; Stage 4, fatty atrophy greater than 50% [24].

2. Treatment

The orthopedic surgeon's community has failed, to the date, to clearly identify which patients would benefit from surgical repair as the primary treatment. Most patients accept an initial attempt of conservative treatment, which is successful in most cases. They undergo a surgical rotator cuff repair if the former fails to provide pain relief and function improvement. Although this strategy is accepted worldwide, it does not provide a definitive solution for the tear, which seldom heals on its own (about 10% of small tears heal, and 10% become smaller). Tear progression is always worrisome as it may lead to non-repairability, arthritis and chronic pain. As a matter of fact, more than 50% of patients with partial tears experience a progression, which is closely correlated with the size of the index tear, and more than half of those with a full-thickness tear will suffer from an increase in the size of the tear, which may be the culprit for an increase in pain and disability. Acute traumatic tears, either in a previously asymptomatic patient or in patients with a previous history of rotator cuff disease yet compensated, with a significant loss of function, are good candidates for surgical repair without unnecessary delays [25–27].

The objective of the orthopedic surgeon, once the surgery is indicated and agreed upon by the patient, is to achieve sound fixation of the cuff to humeral tuberosities. Thorough attention to avoid gap formation is also a must. If the tendon is well fixed close to the bone, healing tissue will develop [28].

Despite some studies that show few differences in pain relief concerning tendon healing or retear, many others have identified a well-healed cuff as the main factor for improved strength and range of motion [28].

2.1 Open vs. arthroscopic

Open rotator cuff repair has been the gold standard when treating cuff tears. However, some concerns about infection and faster recovery have led shoulder surgeons to investigate the use of minimally invasive and arthroscopic technique.

Neviaser et al. retrospectively reviewed a cohort of patients who underwent anterosuperior rotator cuff repair with subscapularis involvement and found no differences in the outcomes between both modalities [29].

Hasler et al. in a prospective, randomized and long-term outcome study comparing open and arthroscopic rotator cuff repair did not document any difference either clinical or radiological. In addition, they did not find any harmful consequence due to transdeltoid mini-open approach [30].

Nazari et al. studied the effects of arthroscopic and mini-open rotator cuff repairs concerning pain and range of motion and did not find significant differences at 3, 6 and 12 months between both techniques [31].

Bayle et al. studied not only clinical outcomes but rotator cuff integrity at 1-year follow-up and did not find differences in a prospective study [32].

Fink Barnes et al. studied patient satisfaction and rotator cuff integrity in a cohort and found better results concerning integrity in the open surgery group. However, no statistical differences were found between both at the end of the study [33].

To sum up, if cost or time is an issue, open rotator cuff surgery is preferred. However, if short-term results are crucial and the patient seeks a faster return to work or sport, the arthroscopic repair is the technique of choice. The patient needs to be advised that both techniques may lead to excellent results and that the community of orthopedic surgeons cannot recommend one over the other if the factors mentioned above are not taken into account.

2.2 Repair techniques

With the advent of open and mini-open techniques, some classic repair techniques were developed. Transosseous sutures were mainly implemented, where bone tunnels are created, and sutures are placed directly through them, allowing for cuff reinsertion, as depicted in **Figure 1**.

A single-row repair is performed by means of anchors, usually one or two, with sutures integrated into them that permit cuff repair, as depicted in **Figure 2**. Single-row techniques are easier to perform arthroscopically, as well as in an open fashion.

Double-row repairs use one or two anchors in a medial row, suturing far from the tendon stump border area and a lateral row, again with one or two anchors, closer to

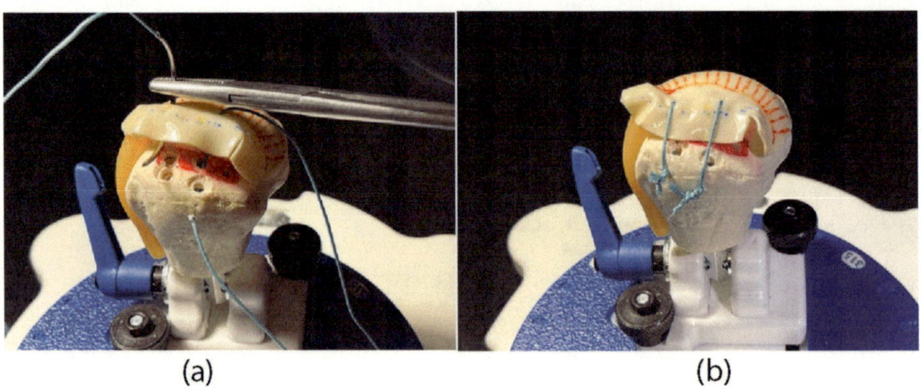

Figure 1.
a. and b. Transosseous repair, usually used in open surgery.

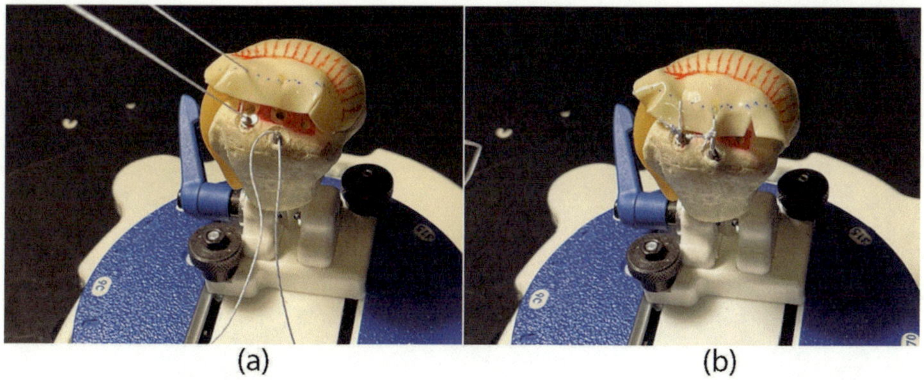

Figure 2.
a. and b. classic single-row repair with two lateral anchors.

the end of the ruptured tendon and the lateral border of the cuff footprint along the tuberosity, as it can be seen in **Figure 3**.

More recent are transosseous equivalent techniques, similar to double-row techniques yet requiring only a medial row and knotless implants laterally (without sutures passing through the tendon laterally but applying those from the medial row against the tendon) (see **Figures 4** and **5**) [28].

2.3 Single vs. double row

Single- and double-row techniques have been compared about their failure loads and gap formation. In an experimental study, Kim et al. and Ma et al. reported significant more load to failure and less gap formation in favor of double row. They also confirmed in vitro that the strain using a double row was a third of that of a single row. However, other studies, such as the one performed by Mazzoca et al., compared both without finding any difference. Finally, a meta-analysis by Hohmann et al. revealed a possible superiority in vitro regarding gap formation and load to failure yet not observed clinically in vivo. Therefore, a superiority of a technique versus the other has not been demonstrated, and the final decision belongs to the orthopedic surgeon

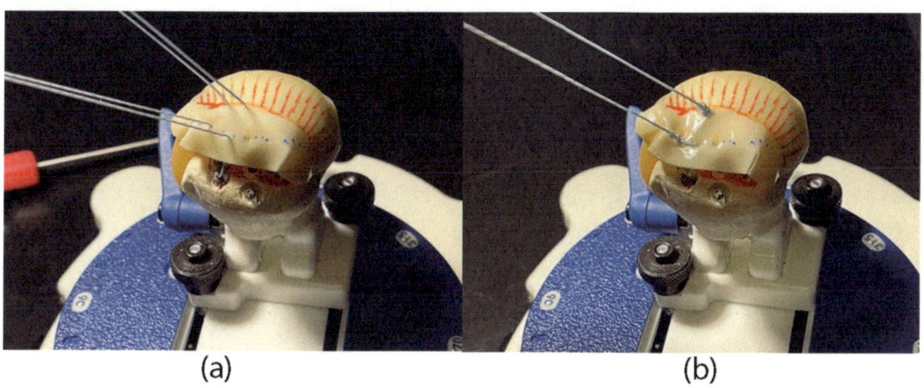

Figure 3.
a. and b. classic double-row configurations. Two anchors medial and two anchors lateral to the footprint with mattress sutures.

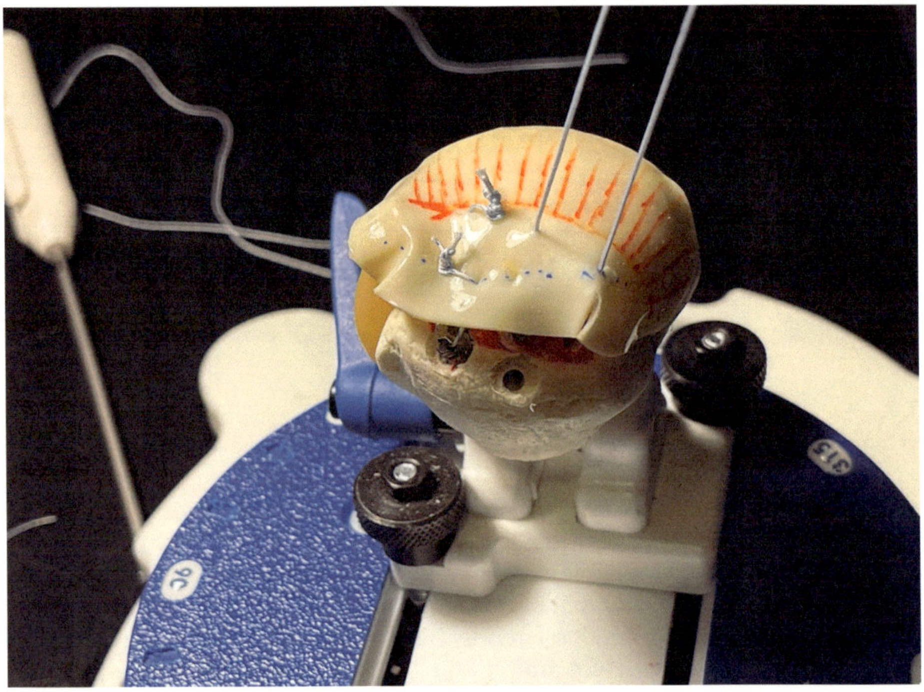

Figure 4.
On the left, a classic double row with independent sutures and anchors. On the right, the medial row sutures have been passed through the cuff, very close to the musculotendinous junction.

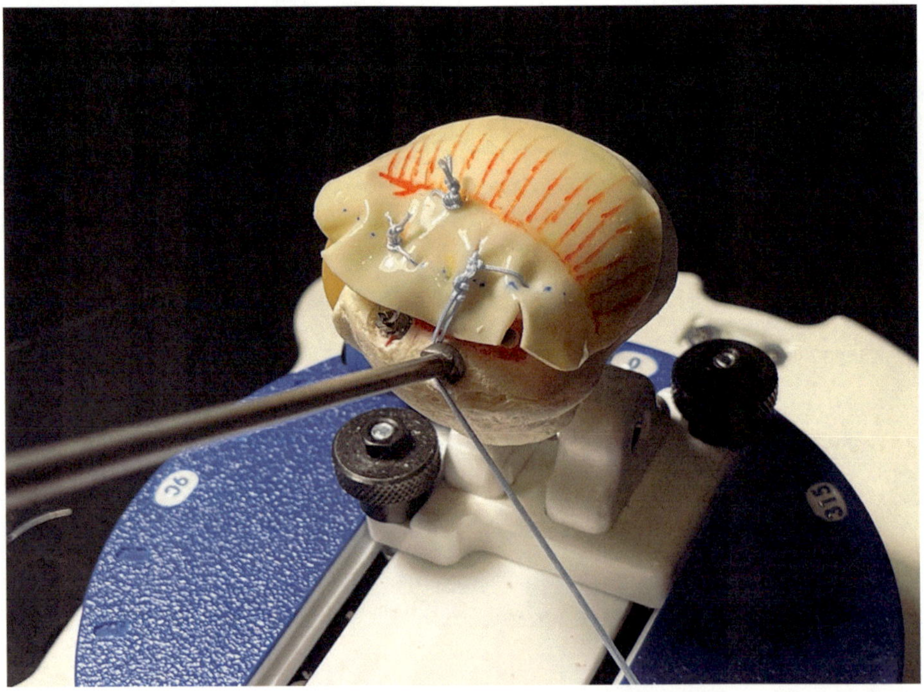

Figure 5.
The medial row mattress sutures, tied, are inserted into the bone, lateral to the footprint, by means of a knotless anchor.

who should analyze factors such as simplicity, skill, cost and time consumption when choosing the right technique for the patient [28, 34–36].

Deveci et al. and Maasse et al. reported that most studies comparing single- and double-row techniques were comparing different constructs and suture configurations, and thus the results obtained are not valid. Most studies used lateral single-row configurations either in vitro or in vivo, and very few a more medial single row avoiding unnecessary tension at the level of the repair (which is a must, especially in large and retracted tears) When a proper, more medial, single-row configuration was used, the results become similar. It is not fair to compare single-row configurations performed poorly and too lateral to modern double-row techniques, and despite that, clinically relevant results have failed to be obtained [37, 38].

2.4 Transsosseous vs. single row

Transosseous repairs are of everyday use during open rotator cuff repair. The use of bony tunnels avoids anchors, which is a significant advantage concerning cost and ease of revision surgery. The former is performed either by employing guides and Kirschner wires or bone needles in the osteoporotic bone. Ahmad et al. and Park et al.compared micromotion in vitro at the footprint interface and concluded that transosseous repair minimizes strain and, therefore, would be advantageous concerning tendon to bone healing. Apreleva et al., in another experimental study, demonstrated that footprint anatomy restoration was superior when using transosseous techniques [39–42].

On the contrary, other authors such as Randelly et al. in a clinical study concluded that single-row and transosseous hardware-free repairs led to the same results concerning pain, function and retear rate at 15 months. However, transosseous repairs might be more cost-effective because they avoid the use of anchors [43].

Same principles apply to partial repairs when comparing transtendon single-row techniques versus double-row suture bridges. Zafra et al. demonstrated that partial tears might be treated with similar results using both techniques [44].

2.5 Transosseous vs. double row

Traditional transosseous repair focuses on restoring cuff footprint and applying pressure on the enthesis (against tuberosity bone). On the contrary, the traditional double row focuses on suturing the tendon medial and lateral in the footprint. Waltrip et al. compared both and demonstrated that a higher stress concentration was found in the latter at the medial anchors and suturing areas, while the former had more significant stress at the tendon to bone interface level. Forces through the tendon to bone enthesis can be beneficial, and on the contrary, forces around the anchors may explain the high recurrence rate and pull-out observed in double-row repairs [28, 45].

2.6 Transosseous equivalent vs. double row

Transosseous equivalent techniques mimic the effect created by traditional transosseous techniques utilizing lateral knotless anchors, which insert the sutures used in the medial row into the lateral cortex of the tuberosity. Hence, this technique mimics the effect of the classic techniques as it adds pressure forces that apply the tendon stump against the bone.

Siskoksy et al., in a cadaveric study, compared load to failure and gap formation using transosseous equivalent and double-row techniques. They concluded that load to failure was higher when using a transosseous equivalent construct. However, gap formation was similar between both [46]. The same conclusion was obtained by Costic et al. in a similar study in cadavers where cyclic loading was applied on the footprint [47].

Park et al. demonstrated in vitro that the pressure exerted by a transosseous equivalent is significantly higher than that observed in double rows. Nevertheless, it remains difficult to know the right amount of pressure or the ischemic effect of an excessive force on the tendon stump [48].

3. The art of the single-row technique

Not all single-row techniques are created equal. Arthroscopic rotator cuff repair emerged in the 1990s, and logically single-row constructs were the first used by shoulder and sports medicine surgeons. Initially, a unique row formed by one or two anchors (placed in the centre of the footprint or lateral to it) was used.

Not all single-row techniques are created equal. Arthroscopic rotator cuff repair emerged in the 1990s, and logically single-row constructs were the first used by shoulder and sports medicine surgeons. Initially, a unique row formed by one or two anchors (placed in the centre of the footprint or lateral to it) was used. Despite initial promising outcomes, the retear rate was undoubtedly worrisome, which explains the subsequent interest in developing double rows or transosseous equivalent techniques.

Complex and more robust suture configurations (such as the Mason-Allen technique) are complicated to replicate arthroscopically.

Simple or mattress sutures, often used arthroscopically, may not be sufficient to hold a rotator cuff with poor-quality tissue to the bone long enough to allow for proper healing. These statements led to a quest to find a better technique by adding anchors and complexity to the repairs. However, it was not until later that some surgeons started to question if a well-performed single row would be sufficient. To do so, a more medial single row started to be used with the rationale behind it that less tension on the rotator cuff would result. This is very useful in the onset of chronic and massive tears where even after proper slide liberation, tendon retraction impedes proper footprint anatomical restoration, as depicted in **Figures 6–9** [49].

Several factors may contribute to the final healing of the rotator cuff tendons to the bone. Among them, mechanical factors such as gap formation, stiffness and strength of the repair, load to failure, repair tension have already been discussed in previous sections of this chapter. However, other factors such as tendon vascularity, footprint coverage and respecting the proper biology of tendon healing are sometimes forgotten [49].

Suture bridge techniques have demonstrated in vitro superior strength, stiffness, less gap formation and more load to failure. However, this comes at the cost of vascularity disruption, high tension at the muscle to tendon junction (which may lead to a tear at this level). Transosseous equivalent techniques enhance the resistance and stability of the repair at the tendon to bone interface; nevertheless, they neglect biology as they create an ischemic environment. As a matter of fact, in vivo studies have failed to demonstrate the superiority of transosseous rotator cuff repair over single-row repair [49, 50].

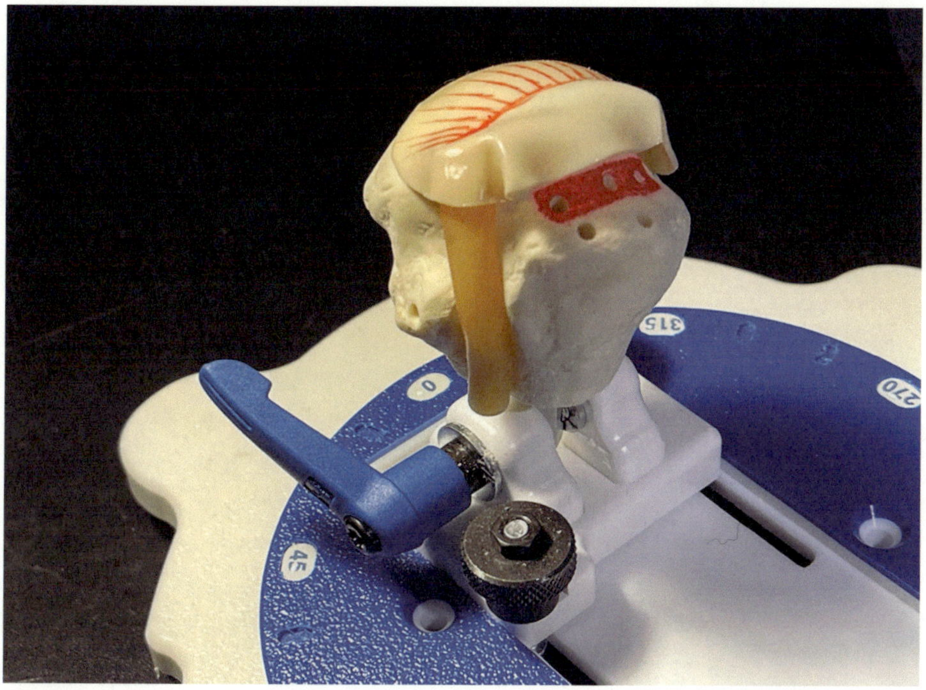

Figure 6.
Classic single row is performed with anchors in a more central or even lateral position in the footprint. Modern single row uses anchors closer to the cartilage, in a more medial position in the footprint (red area).

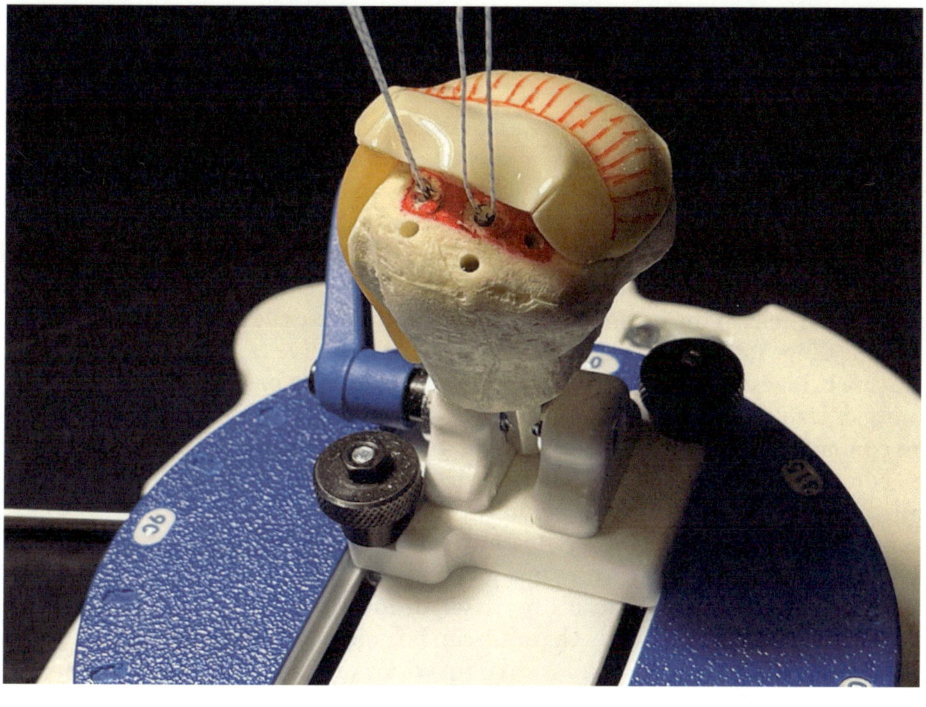

Figure 7.
The number of anchors varies between one and three depending on the size of the tear.

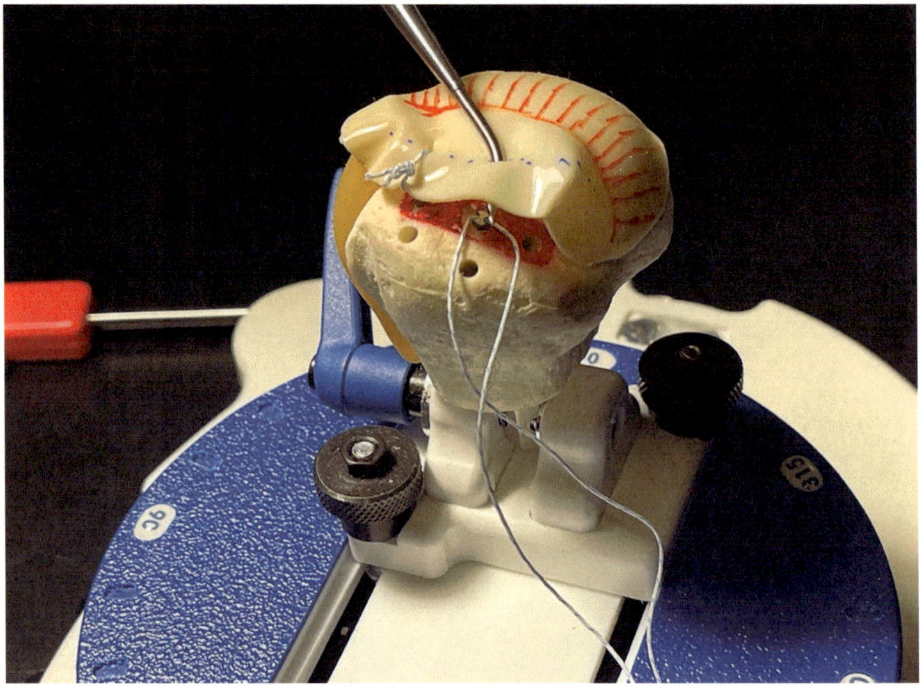

Figure 8.
A modern single-row construct uses sutures that pass about 1 cm medial to the border of the tendon stump. Thus, reducing the tension and minimizing retear rates due to excessive tension or damage to the musculotendinous junction.

In the context of a single-row repair, a more medial row may enhance biology as it adds less loading forces and respects vascularity. However, footprint non-anatomic restoration may arise as a concern. By medializing the anchors in the footprint (not medial to it), a part of the surface may stay uncovered by the tendon stump. Although the real significance of this has not been established, surgeons commonly think anatomic restoration would be superior to a 'leave it alone' strategy. To cope with this problem, creating bone marrow vents through microfracture instruments would promote the formation of a neotendon and fibrocartilage. The benefits of adding mesenchymal cells to the healing area would also increase the chances of the tendon to bone healing. Yamakado et al. concluded in a prospective randomized trial comparing suture bridge configurations and single-row (medially based) repairs that both techniques lead to the same clinical results. They found that incomplete healing was more common in single-row repairs, and on the other hand, medial cuff failure was more common in patients with bridge constructs. However, the differences were not significant from a statistical point of view [49].

Another argument favoring single-row techniques is that excessive medial sutures in the cuff may lead to a myotendinous junction tear. Despite some authors that studied the use of more medial sutures in vitro, advocating for more stability of the construct, it is accepted globally that this can be dangerous as it might come with a rupture at the level of the muscle, ending up with a tendon stump anchored to the tuberosity but without a healthy muscle able to apply traction on it. Therefore, leaving a security distance from the musculotendinous junction of 10 mm is the wiser choice [51, 52].

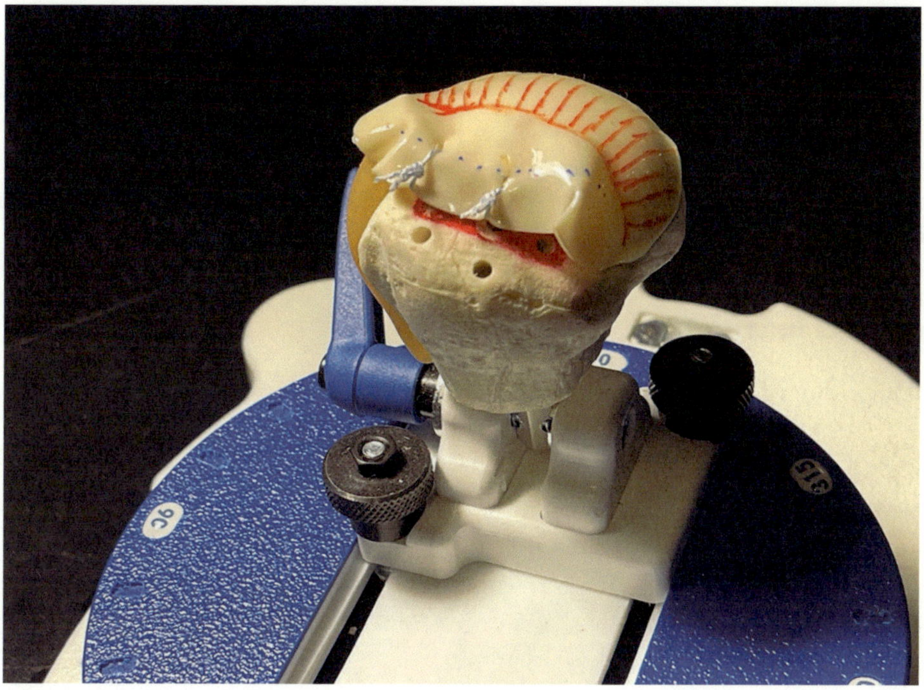

Figure 9.
Final modern single-row construct. Sutures are passed through the tendon far from the musculotendinous junction and far from the border. Less footprint is covered by the cuff when using this technique; however, bone marrow vents, lateral to the footprint, may provide stem cells which will develop a neotendon.

It has also been suggested that a single-row technique mimicking the Masson-Allen suture technique might increase the strength of the repair. Despite some studies confirming that these modifications of the original technique ('modified Mason Allen' or 'massive cuff suture configuration') might increase in vitro the stability of the repair (similar to the original Mason-Allen technique), they have failed to demonstrate a statistical difference or a real relevance clinically. In fact, rotator cuff repairs usually fail at the suture-tissue interface due to poor quality of the latter; therefore, the culprit might not be suture configuration. This the interest in keeping it as simple as possible [53–58].

4. Conclusions

Rotator cuff tear is a common etiology for pain, disability and loss of function that might be considered a burden for some health systems.

Conservative treatment may be adequate for a large number of patients; however, it is utterly crucial to identify patients who would benefit from an acute repair and not to neglect patients who still suffer and do not achieve a satisfactory result employing conservative methods.

The selection of the surgical technique for those patients who require a rotator cuff repair should be guided by the current evidence. It should favor methods that provide the best results for the patient while maintaining simplicity and cost-effectiveness at the proper levels. Therefore, a modern single-row technique with a more medial anchor placement and bone marrow vents in the rotator footprint is probably the technique that balances all the factors mentioned before.

Acknowledgements

The authors would like to thank ASIS Medica for their support in the development of this study.

Conflict of interest

The authors declare no conflict of interest.

Author details

Amhaz Escanlar S.[1]*, Jorge Mora A.[2] and Pino Miguez J.[3]

1 University Hospital Complex, Santiago de Compostela, Spain

2 Reconstructive Surgery, University Hospital Complex, Santiago de Compostela, Spain

3 Pediatric Orthopedics and Spine Surgery, University Hospital Complex, Santiago de Compostela, Spain

*Address all correspondence to: sameramhaz@gmail.com

References

[1] Hantes EM, Chalatsis IG, Mpakagiannis G. Single-row versus double-row repair in rotator cuff tears. In: Surgical Recovery. Rijeka: IntechOpen; 2020

[2] Fehringer EV, Sun J, VanOeveren LS, Keller BK, Matsen FA 3rd. Full-thickness rotator cuff tear prevalence and correlation with function and co-morbidities in patients sixty-five years and older.Journal of Shoulder and Elbow Surgery. 2008 Nov-Dec;**17**(6):881-885. DOI: 10.1016/j.jse.2008.05.039. Epub 2008 Sep 6. PMID: 18774738.

[3] Moosmayer S, Smith H-J, Tariq R, Larmo A. Prevalence and characteristics of asymptomatic tears of the rotator cuff: An ultrasonographic and clinical study. The Journal of Bone and Joint Surgery British Volume. 2009;**91**(2):196-200

[4] Teunis T, Lubberts B, Reilly BT, Ring D. A systematic review and pooled analysis of the prevalence of rotator cuff disease with increasing age. Journal of Shoulder and Elbow Surgery. 2014;**23**(12):1913-1921

[5] Yamaguchi K, Ditsios K, Middleton WD, Hildebolt CF, Galatz LM, Teefey SA. The demographic and morphological features of rotator cuff disease. A comparison of asymptomatic and symptomatic shoulders. The Journal of Bone and Joint Surgery American Volume. 2006;**88**(8):1699-1704

[6] Abate M, Schiavone C, di Carlo L, Salini V. Prevalence of and risk factors for asymptomatic rotator cuff tears in postmenopausal women. Menopause (New York, NY). 2014;**21**(3):275-280

[7] Zumstein MA, Künzler M, Hatta T, Galatz LM, Itoi E. Rotator cuff pathology: State of the art. Journal of ISAKOS: Joint Disorders & Orthopaedic Sports Medicine. 2017;**2**(4):213-221

[8] Keener JD, Galatz LM, Teefey SA, Middleton WD, Steger-May K, Stobbs-Cucchi G, et al. A prospective evaluation of survivorship of asymptomatic degenerative rotator cuff tears. The Journal of Bone and Joint Surgery American Volume. 2015;**97**(2):89-98

[9] Pauly S, Stahnke K, Klatte-Schulz F, Wildemann B, Scheibel M, Greiner S. Do patient age and sex influence tendon cell biology and clinical/radiographic outcomes after rotator cuff repair? The American Journal of Sports Medicine. 2015;**43**(3):549-556

[10] Milgrom C, Schaffler M, Gilbert S, van Holsbeeck M. Rotator-cuff changes in asymptomatic adults. The effect of age, hand dominance and gender. The Journal of Bone and Joint Surgery British Volume. 1995;**77**(2):296-298

[11] Liem D, Buschmann VE, Schmidt C, Gosheger G, Vogler T, Schulte TL, et al. The prevalence of rotator cuff tears: Is the contralateral shoulder at risk? The American Journal of Sports Medicine. 2014;**42**(4):826-830

[12] Yamamoto A, Takagishi K, Osawa T, Yanagawa T, Nakajima D, Shitara H, et al. Prevalence and risk factors of a rotator cuff tear in the general population. Journal of Shoulder and Elbow Surgery. 2010;**19**(1):116-120

[13] Kim KC, Shin HD, Cha SM, Park JY. Repair integrity and functional outcome after arthroscopic conversion to a full-thickness rotator cuff tear: Articular-versus bursal-side partial tears. The American Journal of Sports Medicine. 2014;**42**(2):451-456

[14] Lee TQ. Current biomechanical concepts for rotator cuff repair. Clinics in Orthopedic Surgery. 2013;**5**(2):89-97

[15] Lindley K, Jones GL. Outcomes of arthroscopic versus open rotator cuff repair: A systematic review of the literature. American Journal of Orthopedics (Belle Mead, NJ). 2010;**39**(12):592-600

[16] Neer CS. Anterior acromioplasty for the chronic impingement syndrome in the shoulder: A preliminary report. The Journal of Bone and Joint Surgery American volume. 1972;**54**(1):41-50

[17] Cofield RH. Subscapular muscle transposition for repair of chronic rotator cuff tears. Surgery, Gynecology & Obstetrics. 1982;**154**(5):667-672

[18] Kuhn JE, Dunn WR, Ma B, Wright RW, Jones G, Spencer EE, et al. Interobserver agreement in the classification of rotator cuff tears. The American Journal of Sports Medicine. 2007;**35**(3):437-441

[19] Lädermann A, Burkhart SS, Hoffmeyer P, Neyton L, Collin P, Yates E, et al. Classification of full-thickness rotator cuff lesions: A review. EFORT Open Reviews. 2016;**1**(12):420-430

[20] Ellman H, Kay SP, Wirth M. Arthroscopic treatment of full-thickness rotator cuff tears: 2- to 7-year follow-up study. Arthroscopy: The Journal of Arthroscopic & Related Surgery: Official Publication of the Arthroscopy Association of North America and the International Arthroscopy Association. 1993;**9**(2):195-200

[21] Ellman H. Diagnosis and treatment of incomplete rotator cuff tears. Clinical Orthopaedics and Related Research. 1990;**254**:64-74

[22] Fox JA, Cole BJ, Romeo AA, Meininger AK, Williams JM, Glenn RE, et al. Articular cartilage thickness of the humeral head: An anatomic study. Orthopedics. 2008;**31**(3):216

[23] Patte D. Classification of rotator cuff lesions. Clinical Orthopaedics and Related Research. 1990;**254**:81-86

[24] Goutallier D, Postel JM, Bernageau J, Lavau L, Voisin MC. Fatty muscle degeneration in cuff ruptures. Pre- and Postoperative Evaluation by CT scan. Clinical Orthopaedics and Related Research. 1994;**304**:78-83

[25] Mall NA, Kim HM, Keener JD, Steger-May K, Teefey SA, Middleton WD, et al. Symptomatic progression of asymptomatic rotator cuff tears: A prospective study of clinical and sonographic variables. The Journal of Bone and Joint Surgery American volume. 2010;**92**(16):2623-2633

[26] Millett PJ, Warth RJ, Dornan GJ, Lee JT, Spiegl UJ. Clinical and structural outcomes after arthroscopic single-row versus double-row rotator cuff repair: A systematic review and meta-analysis of level I randomized clinical trials. Journal of Shoulder and Elbow Surgery. 2014;**23**(4):586-597

[27] Gilotra M, O'Brien MJ, Savoie FH. Arthroscopic rotator cuff repair: Indication and technique. Instructional Course Lectures. 2016;**65**:83-92

[28] Cole BJ, ElAttrache NS, Anbari A. Arthroscopic rotator cuff repairs: An anatomic and biomechanical rationale for different suture-anchor repair configurations. Arthroscopy: The Journal of Arthroscopic and Related Surgery. 2007;**23**(6):662-669

[29] Neviaser AS, Charen DA, Cotter JM, Harrison AK, Cagle PJ, Flatow EL.

Retrospective review of open and arthroscopic repair of anterosuperior rotator cuff tears with subscapularis involvement: A single surgeon's experience. Journal of Shoulder and Elbow Surgery. 2020;**29**(5):893-897

[30] Hasler A, Beeler S, Götschi T, Catanzaro S, Jost B, Gerber C. No difference in long-term outcome between open and arthroscopic rotator cuff repair: A prospective, randomized study. JSES International. 2020;**4**(4):818-825

[31] Nazari G, MacDermid JC, Bryant D, Dewan N, Athwal GS. Effects of arthroscopic vs. mini-open rotator cuff repair on function, pain & range of motion. A systematic review and meta-analysis. PLoS One. 2019 Oct 31;**14**(10):e0222953. DOI: 10.1371/journal.pone.0222953. PMID: 31671101; PMCID: PMC6822715.

[32] Bayle X, Pham TT, Faruch M, Gobet A, Mansat P, Bonnevialle N. No difference in outcome for open versus arthroscopic rotator cuff repair: A prospective comparative trial. Archives of Orthopaedic and Trauma Surgery. 2017;**137**(12):1707-1712

[33] Barnes LA, Kim HM, Caldwell JM, Buza J, Ahmad CS, Bigliani LU, Levine WN. Satisfaction, function and repair integrity after arthroscopic versus mini-open rotator cuff repair. Bone Joint J. 2017 Feb;**99**(2):245-249. DOI: 10.1302/0301-620X.99B2.BJJ-2016-0055.R1. PMID: 28148668.

[34] Ma CB, Comerford L, Wilson J, Puttlitz CM. Biomechanical evaluation of arthroscopic rotator cuff repairs: Double-row compared with single-row fixation. The Journal of Bone and Joint Surgery American Volume. 2006;**88**(2):403-410

[35] Mazzocca AD, Millett PJ, Guanche CA, Santangelo SA, Arciero RA. Arthroscopic single-row versus double-row suture anchor rotator cuff repair. The American Journal of Sports Medicine. 2005;**33**(12):1861-1868

[36] Kim DH, Elattrache NS, Tibone JE, Jun B-J, DeLaMora SN, Kvitne RS, et al. Biomechanical comparison of a single-row versus double-row suture anchor technique for rotator cuff repair. The American Journal of Sports Medicine. 2006;**34**(3):407-414

[37] Deveci A. What is wrong in comparison of single- and double-row repairs in rotator cuff tears? European Journal of Orthopaedic Surgery and Traumatology. 2019;**29**:1589-1590

[38] Maassen NH, Somerson JS. A majority of single versus double-row rotator cuff repair comparisons fail to consider modern single-row techniques: A systematic review. JBJS Reviews. 2020;**8**(5):e0203

[39] Park MC, Cadet ER, Levine WN, Bigliani LU, Ahmad CS. Tendon-to-bone pressure distributions at a repaired rotator cuff footprint using transosseous suture and suture anchor fixation techniques. The American Journal of Sports Medicine. 2005;**33**(8):1154-1159

[40] Cummins CA, Appleyard RC, Strickland S, Haen P-S, Chen S, Murrell GAC. Rotator cuff repair: An ex vivo analysis of suture anchor repair techniques on initial load to failure. Arthroscopy: The Journal of Arthroscopic & Related Surgery: Official Publication of the Arthroscopy Association of North America and the International Arthroscopy Association. 2005;**21**(10):1236-1241

[41] Apreleva M, Ozbaydar M, Fitzgibbons PG, Warner JJ. Rotator cuff tears: the effect of the reconstruction method on three-dimensional repair site area. Arthroscopy. 2002

May-Jun;**18**(5):519-526. DOI: 10.1053/jars.2002.32930. PMID: 11987064.

[42] Ahmad CS, Stewart AM, Izquierdo R, Bigliani LU. Tendon-bone interface motion in transosseous suture and suture anchor rotator cuff repair techniques. The American Journal of Sports Medicine. 2005;**33**(11):1667-1671

[43] Ryu RKN. Arthroscopic transosseous suture repair and single-row anchor fixation for rotator cuff lesions did not differ for pain, function, or rotator-cuff integrity at 15 months. The Journal of Bone and Joint Surgery. American Volume. 2017;**99**:1943

[44] Zafra M, Uceda P, Muñoz-Luna F, Muñoz-López RC, Font P. Arthroscopic repair of partial-thickness articular surface rotator cuff tears: Single-row transtendon technique versus double-row suture bridge (transosseous equivalent) fixation: Results from a prospective randomized study. Archives of Orthopaedic and Trauma Surgery [Internet]. 2020;**140**(8):1065-1071. Available from: http://www.ncbi.nlm.nih.gov/pubmed/32170453

[45] Waltrip RL, Zheng N, Dugas JR, Andrews JR. Rotator cuff repair. A biomechanical comparison of three techniques. Am J Sports Med. 2003 Jul-Aug;**31**(4):493-497. DOI: 10.1177/03635465030310040301. PMID: 12860534.

[46] Siskosky MJ, ElAttrache NS, Chu E, Tibone JE, Lee TQ. Biomechanical evaluation of the "transosseous equivalent"rotator cuff repair technique using the PushLock for lateralfixation compared to the double-row technique. In: Presented at the Annual Meeting of the American Academy of OrthopaedicSurgeons, San Diego, CA, February 14-18. 2007

[47] Costic RS, Brucker PU, Smolinski PJ, Gilbertson LG, Ro-dosky MW. Arthroscopic double row anchor repair of fullthickness rotator cuff tear: Footprint restoration and biome-chanical properties. In: Presented at the Annual Meeting of the Orthopaedic Research Society, Chicago, IL, March 19-22. 2006

[48] Park MC, ElAttrache NS, Tibone JE, Ahmad CS, Jun BJ, Lee TQ. Footprint contact biomechanics for a new arthroscopictransosseous-equivalent rotator cuff repair technique com-pared to a double-row technique arthroscopic rotator cuffrepair. In: Presented at the Annual Meeting of the American Academy of Orthopaedic Surgeons, Chicago, IL, March 22-26. 2006

[49] Yamakado K. Two techniques for treating medium-sized supraspinatus tears: The medially based single-row technique and the suture bridge technique. JBJS Essential Surgical Techniques. 2021 Jun 8;**11**(2):e20.00004. DOI: 10.2106/JBJS.ST.20.00004. PMID: 34277130; PMCID: PMC8280021.

[50] Plachel F, Siegert P, Rüttershoff K, Thiele K, Akgün D, Moroder P, et al. Long-term results of arthroscopic rotator cuff repair: A follow-up study comparing single-row versus double-row fixation techniques. American Journal of Sports Medicine. 2020;**48**(7):1568-1574

[51] Virk MS, Bruce B, Hussey KE, Thomas JM, Luthringer TA, Shewman EF, et al. Biomechanical performance of medial row suture placement relative to the musculotendinous junction in transosseous equivalent suture bridge double-row rotator cuff repair. Arthroscopy: The Journal of Arthroscopic and Related Surgery. 2017;**33**(2):242-250

[52] Barber FA. Editorial commentary: Musculotendinous junction mattress sutures are inefficient. Arthroscopy: The Journal of Arthroscopic and Related Surgery. 2017;**33**:251-253

[53] Meisel AF, Henninger HB, Barber FA, Getelman MH. Biomechanical comparison of standard and linked single-row rotator cuff repairs in a human cadaver model. Arthroscopy: The Journal of Arthroscopic and Related Surgery. 2017;**33**(5):938-944

[54] Baleani M, Ohman C, Guandalini L, Rotini R, Giavaresi G, Traina F, et al. Comparative study of different tendon grasping techniques for arthroscopic repair of the rotator cuff. Clinical Biomechanics (Bristol, Avon). 2006;**21**(8):799-803

[55] Galatz LM, Ball CM, Teefey SA, Middleton WD, Yamaguchi K. The outcome and repair integrity of completely arthroscopically repaired large and massive rotator cuff tears. The Journal of Bone and Joint Surgery American Volume. 2004;**86**(2):219-224

[56] Wetzler MJ. Editorial commentary: Belt and suspenders—Linked single-row rotator cuff repair. Arthroscopy: The Journal of Arthroscopic and Related Surgery. 2017;**33**:945

[57] Noyes MP, Lederman E, Adams CR, Denard PJ. Triple-loaded suture anchors versus a knotless rip stop construct in a single-row rotator cuff repair model. Arthroscopy: The Journal of Arthroscopic and Related Surgery. 2018;**34**(5):1414-1420

[58] Noyes MP, Ladermann A, Denard PJ. Functional outcome and healing with a load-sharing rip-stop repair compared with a single-row repair for large and massive rotator cuff tears. Arthroscopy: The Journal of Arthroscopic and Related Surgery. 2019;**35**(8):2295-2300

Chapter 3

Frozen Shoulder: Symptoms, Causes, Diagnosis, and Treatment

Simona Maria Carmignano

Abstract

Frozen shoulder, or adhesive capsulitis, is a condition caused by impaired soft tissues and the articular capsule of the shoulder. Although the precise etiology remains unclear, recent evidence identifies elevated serum cytokine levels as part of the process. It is characterized by an insidious and progressive loss of active and passive mobility in the glenohumeral joint presumably due to capsular contracture. Several treatments are recognized and utilized to reduce pain and improve range-of-motion faster than the disease's natural history course. The chapter aims to spread knowledge about this often-misunderstood pathology and to highlight the role of the rehabilitative therapeutic approach.

Keywords: shoulder, rehabilitation, pain, physical therapy, complementary therapy, physiotherapy

1. Introduction

Frozen shoulder, or adhesive capsulitis, is a condition caused by impaired soft tissues and the articular capsule of the shoulder. Primary frozen shoulder is common, and it is characterized by debilitating conditions. The prevalence is between 2% and 5% that increasing to 10–38% in patients with diabetes and thyroid disease. The age of patients is commonly between 40 and 65 years old, and the incidence appears higher in females than males [1–3]. It may also occur after trauma or in association with other joint diseases, as acromioclavicular osteoarthritis, which is referred to as a secondary frozen shoulder [4].

2. Frozen shoulder: clinical definition

Codman defined frozen shoulder as a clinical condition that can hardly be defined, it is complicated to enclose it in a single pathological mechanism, and therefore, even less easy to define its treatment. Instead, the term "adhesive capsulitis" was introduced by Neviaser [5] to describe a tissue inflammation condition and subsequent fibrosis involving the articular capsule of the shoulder. In addition, the definition of "frozen" shoulder refers to pain and immobility correlation. Lack of function causes the capsule to thicken, making it even more difficult to move. Therefore the functional expression of pathology defines the term "frozen."

Frozen shoulder is characterized by an insidious and progressive loss of active and passive mobility in the glenohumeral joint presumably due to capsular contracture.

Frozen shoulder can be classified as primary or secondary. Primary idiopathic frozen shoulder can be often associated with other diseases, such as diabetes mellitus, thyroid diseases, and Parkinson's disease. Secondary adhesive capsulitis can occur after trauma or immobilization. Frozen shoulder is estimated to affect 2–5% of the general population. A patient who experiments with this pathology can be significantly painful and disabling for some months. It most commonly affects those in their fourth to sixth decades of life and more often occurs in women than in men [6].

3. Frozen shoulder: pathophysiology

The pathophysiological mechanism underlying the pathology remains poorly understood. Scientific literature shows a correlation with elevated serum cytokine levels [7]. Although the precise pathophysiology remains unclear, recent evidence identifies elevated serum levels of cytokines as part of the process. Cytokines are polypeptide, non-antigen-specific mediators that act as communication signals between immune system cells and between them and different organs and tissues. Elevated cytokine levels appear predominantly involved in the cellular mechanisms of inflammation and fibrosis sustained in the primary and some secondary frozen shoulder. Bunker et al. [8] defined that a mild lesional event would trigger an inflammatory response that results in excessive production of fibroblasts, which release type I and type III collagen. Fibroblasts differentiate into myofibroblasts, causing the newly deposited type III collagen to contract. This would result in an imbalance between the inflammatory phase and the remodeling underlying the fibrosis.

Rodeo et al. [9] described pathological processes like inflammation and fibrosis: synovial hyperplasia determines a decrease of vascularity. This phenomenon leads to fibrosis in the sub-synovium and synovium of capsular tissue. This condition could be the expression of an immune response [10]. Other studies have shown that frozen shoulder is associated with a dense collagen matrix containing fibroblasts and myofibroblasts, suggestive of a fibrotic process [9, 11–13]. Furthermore, the component of the immune system that is activated is represented by B lymphocytes, mast cells, and macrophages. Several studies have suggested the immune response overlaps with inflammatory synovitis, leading to capsular fibrosis in the later stages [5, 14].

There are many etiopathological hypotheses, and all studies suggest that both inflammation and fibrosis of the joint capsule are regulated by cytokines, growth factors, MMPs, and immune cells. The results of the next studies will provide the control mechanisms of FS and identify new therapeutic targets to identify its treatment [14–16].

4. Frozen shoulder: symptoms

Patients typically demonstrate a characteristic history, clinical presentation, and recovery. Clinical syndromes include pain, a limited range of motion (ROM), and muscle weakness from disuse [17].

The pain has a typical course involving the entire shoulder up to the insertion of the deltoid muscle. The patient reports difficulty sleeping on the affected side and

DOI: http://dx.doi.org/10.5772/intechopen.102117

difficulty in active movement. Clinical examination shows atrophy of the spinate, restriction on passive mobilization, with painful and limited elevation and external rotation.

Pain is localized in the shoulder (in the deltoid region), sometimes in the arm with functional limitation. In patients who have been in pain for a long time, may present medial to the scapula. This happens because incorrect movements of the scapulothoracic are established to compensate for the limitation of the glenohumeral joint [18].

Neviaser et al. [19] elaborated on the natural history of frozen shoulder and distinguished the following stages:

- Stage 1: It is defined as a pre-adhesive stage. It is characterized by erythematous joint inflammation and mild pain in the most extreme degrees of movement. It is often misunderstood because it has a similar clinical presentation to the impingement of the rotator cuff.

- Stage 2. It is the acute–adhesive stage. Patients complain of severe pain up to almost the last degree of movement of the joint. An inflammatory process with thickening of the synovium and change of connective tissue is highlighted.

- Stage 3. Fibrotic or “frozen” stage. At this stage, fibrosis is characteristic of the presence of more mature adhesions. The pain becomes less intense and joint stiffness becomes prevalent.

- Stage 4. At this stage, the restriction on movement remains but without synovitis. In fact, it is defined as the “thawing” phase. Patients present painless stiffness and movement typically improves by remodeling (**Figure 1**).

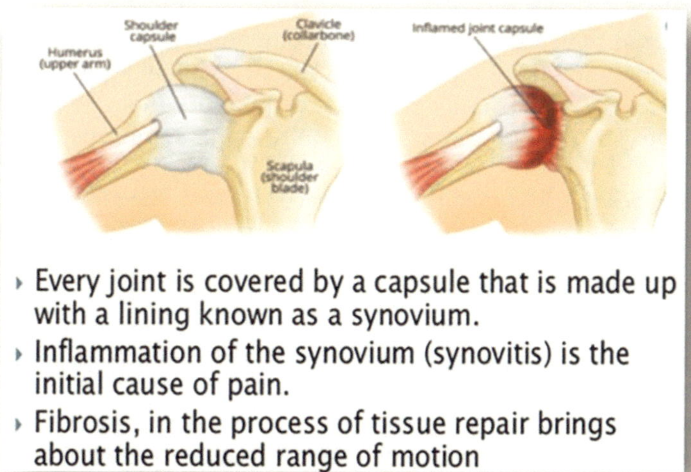

Figure 1.
Natural history of frozen shoulder.

5. Diagnosis

5.1 Clinical diagnosis

Primary frozen shoulder is essentially a clinical diagnosis. Frozen shoulder is characterized by an insidious and progressive loss of active and passive mobility in the glenohumeral joint presumably due to capsular contracture. Patients typically demonstrate a characteristic history, clinical presentation, and recovery. Clinical syndromes include pain, a limited range of motion (ROM), and muscle weakness from disuse [20]. To carry out the clinical examination of the shoulder it is necessary to observe the neck and evaluate through a functional examination if the pain comes from the cervical spine. Subsequently, following the standard shoulder examination protocol, it is necessary to proceed with the inspection of the shoulder. Observe if there are scars, reduced Tropism of rotator cuff/deltoid, bone landmarks, and spinal and scapular alignment. People with frozen shoulders have a limited range of both active and passive motion. Next, proceed to palpation to rule out acromioclavicular-induced pain. Following this, proceed with an assessment of shoulder range of motion (ROM). There are four movements that are useful in the examination—flexion, abduction, internal rotation, and external rotation. Flexion , abduction and internal rotation are evaluated with active and passive mobilization, while external rotation is evaluated only with passive mobilization [21].

Shoulder pain appears slowly and radiates to the insertion of the deltoid. The patient reports inability to sleep on the affected side, limitation to active movement, and painful elevation of the shoulder. Progressively atrophy of the spinate appears.

Imaging studies are not necessary for the diagnosis of adhesive shoulder capsulitis but may be helpful to rule out other causes of a painful and stiff shoulder. Usually, resistance in the last degrees of movement is described, this sensation is defined as firm and "leathery." During the examination the pain is prevalent, the patient cannot get to the point where even the examiner would feel the resistance. Therefore it is most frequently described as a feeling of "empty" end [22].

5.2 Evaluation scale

It should be used to validate functional outcome measures, such as the disabilities of the arm, shoulder, and hand (DASH), the American Shoulder and Elbow Surgeons shoulder scale (ASES), or the Shoulder Pain and Disability Index (SPADI). The DASH questionnaire consists of 30 questions that inquire about symptoms and functions of the upper limbs.

Table 1 describes the 30 items that are carried out with the application of the scale. DASH investigates the severity of pain, activity-related pain, tingling, weakness, and stiffness (five items), and the effect of the upper limb problem on social activities, work, sleep, and self-image (four items). These provide a single main score, the DASH function/symptoms (DASH-FS) score, which is basically a summation of the responses on a one-to-five scale, after transformation to a zero (no disability) to 100 (severe disability) scale [23].

The shoulder and elbow surgeons shoulder scale (ASES) is a physician assessment section that includes physical examination and documentation of a range of motion, strength, and instability, and demonstration of specific physical signs. No score is derived for this section of the instrument. The patient self-evaluation section has 11 items that can be used to generate a score. These are divided into two areas—pain (one item) and function (10 items) (**Table 2**).

Dash questionnaire					
Difficulty	**No**	**Mild**	**Moderate**	**Severe**	**Unable**
1. Open a tight or new jar	1	2	3	4	5
2. Write	1	2	3	4	5
3. Turn a key	1	2	3	4	5
4. Prepare a meal	1	2	3	4	5
5. Push open a heavy door	1	2	3	4	5
6. Place an object on a shelf above your head	1	2	3	4	5
7. Do heavy household chores (e.g., wash walls, wash floors)	1	2	3	4	5
8. Garden or do yard work	1	2	3	4	5
9. Make a bed	1	2	3	4	5
10. Carry a shopping bag or briefcase	1	2	3	4	5
11. Carry a heavy object (over 10 lbs)	1	2	3	4	5
12. Change a light bulb overhead	1	2	3	4	5
13. Wash or blow-dry your hair	1	2	3	4	5
14. Wash your back	1	2	3	4	5
15. Put on a pullover sweater	1	2	3	4	5
16. Use a knife to cut food	1	2	3	4	5
17. Recreational activities that require little effort (e.g., card playing, knitting, etc.)	1	2	3	4	5
18. Recreational activities in which you take some force or impact through your arm, shoulder, or hand (e.g., golf, hammering, tennis, etc.)	1	2	3	4	5
19. Recreational activities in which you move your arm freely (e.g., playing frisbee, badminton, etc.)	1	2	3	4	5
20. Manage transportation needs (getting from one place to another)	1	2	3	4	5
21. Sexual activities	1	2	3	4	5
Disabilities					
	Not at all	**Slightly**	**Moderately**	**Quite a bit**	**Extremely**
22. During the past week, to what extent has your arm, shoulder, or hand problem interfered with your normal social activities with family, friends, neighbors, or groups?	1	2	3	4	5
	Not limited at all	**Slightly limited**	**Moderately limited**	**Very limited**	**Unable**
23. During the past week, were you limited in your work or other regular daily activities as a result of your arm, shoulder, or hand problem?	1	2	3	4	5

Dash questionnaire					
Difficulty	**No**	**Mild**	**Moderate**	**Severe**	**Unable**
Severity symptoms in the last week					
	None	**Mild**	**Moderate**	**Severe**	**Extreme**
24. Arm, shoulder, or hand pain.	1	2	3	4	5
25. Arm, shoulder. or hand pain when you performed any specific activity	1	2	3	4	5
26. Tingling (pins and needles) in your arm, shoulder, or hand	1	2	3	4	5
27. Weakness in your arm, shoulder, or hand	1	2	3	4	5
28. Stiffness in your arm, shoulder, or hand	1	2	3	4	5
Difficulty	**No**	**Mild**	**Moderate**	**Severe**	**So much-I cannot sleep**
29. During the past week, how much difficulty have you had sleeping because of the pain in your arm, shoulder, or hand?	1	2	3	4	5
	Strongly disagree	**Disagree**	**Neither agree nor disagree**	**Agree**	**Strongly agree**
30. I feel less capable, less confident, or less useful because of my arm, shoulder, or hand problem	1	2	3	4	5
Work module (optional)					
This part of the scale is about the impact on working skills (including doing housework). These are four questions that concern five levels of difficulty in using the shoulder during work activities					
Sports/performing arts module (optional)					
This part of the scale is about the impact of playing musical instruments or sport or both. These are four questions that concern five levels of difficulty in using the shoulder during work activities					

Table 1.
Disabilities of the arm, shoulder, and hand (DASH).

The final score is tabulated by multiplying the pain score (maximum 10) by 5 (therefore total possible 50) and the cumulative activity score (maximum 30) by 5/3 (therefore, a total possible 50) for a total of 100 [24].

The Shoulder Pain and Disability Index (SPADI) is a self-administered questionnaire that consists of two dimensions, one for pain and the other for functional activities. The pain dimension consists of five questions regarding the severity of an individual's pain [25].

5.3 Diagnostic imaging

Radiographic examination is carried out to make the differential diagnosis and exclude other pathologies, for example, calcific tendinitis, rupture of the rotator cuff, arthritis of the glenohumeral, and acromioclavicular joint or a neoplastic process. In

Shoulder and elbow surgeons shoulder scale (ASES)		
1. Usual work		
2. Usual sport/leisure activity?		
3. Do you have shoulder pain at night?	Yes	No
4. Do you take pain killers, such as paracetamol (acetaminophen), diclofenac, or ibuprofen?	Yes	No
5. Do you take strong pain killers, such as codeine, tramadol, or morphine?	Yes	No
6. How many pills do you take on an average day?		
7. Intensity of pain?	Visual analog scales (VAS)—from **10** (pain as bad as it can be) to **0** (No pain at all)	
8. Is it difficult for you to put on a coat?	1. Unable to do 2. Very difficult to do 3. Somewhat difficult 4. Not difficult	
9. Is it difficult for you to sleep on the affected side?	1. Unable to do 2. Very difficult to do 3. Somewhat difficult 4. Not difficult	
10. Is it difficult for you to wash your back/do up bra?	1. Unable to do 2. Very difficult to do 3. Somewhat difficult 4. Not difficult	
11. Is it difficult for you to manage toileting?	1. Unable to do 2. Very difficult to do 3. Somewhat difficult 4. Not difficult	

Table 2.
Shoulder and elbow surgeons shoulder scale (ASES).

patients with frozen shoulder radiographic examination is normal, however, osteopenia of the humerus head may be an indirect sign [26].

Ultrasound is an essential tool for diagnosing shoulder disorders. However, the role of ultrasound in assessing and diagnosing adhesive capsulitis has not been fully studied. Sonography had high diagnostic accuracy for the diagnosis of adhesive capsulitis using a combination of parameters, such as coracohumeral ligament (CHL) thickness, rotator interval (RI) thickness, and hypervascularity, axillary recess (AR) thickness [27, 28].

Several studies have shown that the CHL is thickened and stiffened in adhesive capsulitis on ultrasound [29–31]. Other researches correlate AR thickening as a key diagnostic finding of adhesive capsulitis [32] and approximately the AR cutoff value for adhesive capsulitis diagnosis was 4 mm [28].

RI vascularity is a sign of adhesive capsulitis, but controversy remains in the literature about hypervascularity of the RI in adhesive capsulitis [33].

Magnetic resonance imaging (MRI) and magnetic resonance angiography (MRA) may reveal thickening of capsular and pericapsular tissues as well as a contracted glenohumeral joint space. Sliding movement of the supraspinatus tendon [34].

Arthrography is rarely indicated in the diagnosis of frozen shoulder syndrome. It is an invasive procedure that is painful and costly and does not necessarily provide diagnostic insight but it may be associated with a therapeutic articular injection of corticosteroids as a therapeutic intervention [35].

6. Treatments

The goal of the treatment of adhesive capsulitis is to restore the shoulder to a painless and functional joint [36, 37].

6.1 Pharmacological treatment

Initial treatment is aimed at reducing inflammation and pain. Analgesic and anti-inflammatory drugs are used. Aspirin and paracetamol are the most used and with fewer side effects, the dosage is similar to that used in osteoarthritis. Among the nonsteroidal anti-inflammatory drugs (NSAIDs) the most commonly used are ibuprofen, which has the lowest incidence of side effects, naproxen, and diclofenac [38].

Corticosteroids (for which the generic term "steroids" is usually used) strongly suppress all stages of acute and chronic inflammation. In relation to frozen shoulders, they may be injected intra-articularly (directly into the joint) or taken orally. Intra-articular injections of corticosteroids are the most used method. Corticosteroid intra-articular injections demonstrate short-term (4–6 weeks) benefits. Literature reported a moderate effect of corticosteroid injections on pain, external rotation ROM, and disability at 6 weeks, and only small effects after 12 weeks [39, 40]. Corticosteroid injections have been shown to be as effective as exercise for treating frozen shoulder, particularly when provided in the early stages of the pathology. Blanchard et al. [41] suggested that corticosteroid injections have a greater effect when compared to physical therapy when utilized within the first 6 weeks of treatment, although these differences diminished over time.

The injection of sodium hyaluronate (defined as distension or hydrodilation therapy) into the glenohumeral joint for the treatment of adhesive capsulitis results in an improvement in pain and range of motion, similar to the effects of corticosteroid injection but with fewer side effects. Hyaluronic acid has anti-inflammatory properties and it is similar the synovial fluid that occurs naturally in the joints. It works by acting like a lubricant and shock absorber in the joints and helps the joints to work properly [42].

These lubricating effects of hyaluronate have led to use in orthopedic surgery as well, via prevention of adhesion formation after both wrist and finger flexor tendon repair [43]. Thus, extrapolation to the treatment of stiff shoulder and adhesive capsulitis has demonstrated success and improvements in range of motion, pain, and function.

6.1.1 Physical therapy

6.1.1.1 Ultrasound

A common clinical practice among physical therapists is the use of ultrasound prior to capsular and soft tissue stretching techniques based upon its thermal and mechanical effects. Ultrasound is used to manage several soft-tissue conditions, such as tendinitis, bursitis, and muscle spasm; reabsorb calcium deposits in soft tissue; and reduce joint contractures, pain, and scar tissue. Used in conjunction with hot packs, muscle spasms and muscle guarding may be reduced [44]. The effect of ultrasound therapy at a frequency of 1 MHz, unlike the hot pack that produces surface heating, is a heating in the deeper tissues due to the increase in blood flow resulting in an analgesic muscle relaxant effect and wash out of pain mediators. Ultrasound therapy is used in association with the electric current that produces a modulation of muscle tone or further modulates pain. Robertson et al. [45] reported the usage of ultrasound therapy (UST) clinically in the rehabilitation of patients with frozen shoulders. Direct contact is the most common method that therapist applies ultrasound. It consists in the application of a transducer that is pressed gently into conductive gel and against the skin.

It is recommended that ultrasound be applied in a pulsed mode at low intensity (0.5–1.0 W/cm^2) during the acute phase of inflammation to minimize the risk of aggravating the condition and to accelerate recovery, and that continuous ultrasound at high enough intensity to increase tissue temperature be applied in combination with stretching to assist in the resolution of chronic phase, only if the problem is accompanied by soft tissue shortening [46–48]. In a guideline it is reported that therapeutic ultrasound (US) was effective in the treatment of calcific tendonitis of the shoulder, there was no evidence that it was beneficial for other forms of shoulder pain (e.g., capsulitis, bursitis, tendonitis) [49].

The use of ultrasound therapy is indicated as a treatment for the painful phase of adhesive capsulitis and is indicated in the literature alone or in therapy with other therapies (stretching, mobilization, transcutaneous electrotherapy, and laser therapy) with a type B degree of evidence (there is research-based evidence to support the recommendation) [50]. Other studies have shown efficacy not superior to other therapies [51].

6.1.1.2 Transcutaneous electrical nerve stimulation (TENS)

TENS consists of low-frequency electrical pulses (generated by a small, portable unit) transmitted to the tissues through electrodes on the skin. The pulses stimulate peripheral nerves in such a way as to suppress the perception of pain. TENS therapy determines analgesia by different mechanisms—by causing interactions between types of nerve fibers, resulting in a "block" on the transmission of pain signals to the brain; or by releasing hormones that block pain receptors in the central nervous system. The effects of transcutaneous electrical nerve stimulation (TENS) for the treatment of adhesive capsulitis seem to be superior in comparison to stretching exercise [52].

6.1.1.3 Electromagnetic therapy

Electromagnetic fields (EMFs) provide a noninvasive, safe, and easy method to treat pain with respect to musculoskeletal diseases. Magnetic field therapy was applied to promote bone healing, treat osteoarthritis and inflammatory diseases of the musculoskeletal system, alleviate pain, enhance healing of ulcers, and reduce spasticity [53, 54]. This mechanism could promote the resolution of pain by accelerating the removal of inflammatory substances. PEMF stimulates chondrocyte proliferation, differentiation, and extracellular matrix synthesis through the release of anabolic morphogens, such as bone morphogenetic proteins and anti-inflammatory cytokines [55].

Pulsed electromagnetic field (PEMF) therapy has been reported to produce anti-inflammatory and bone-healing effects, but it is unclear whether—it is more or less effective than placebo, or whether other electrotherapy modalities are an effective adjunct to exercise for the treatment of frozen shoulder.

6.1.1.4 Extracorporeal shock wave therapy (ESWT)

ESWT has been recently receiving attention for the treatment of the frozen shoulder. Extracorporeal shock waves therapy (ESWT) represents a valid tool for a wide range of disorders, both in orthopedics and rehabilitative medicine (tendon pathologies, bone healing disturbances, vascular bone diseases), but also in dermatology and vulnology (wound healing disturbances, ulcers, painful scars), neurology (spastic hypertonia and related disturbances), some andrologic disturbances (induratio penis plastica and erectyle disfunctions), and cardiology (in relation to ischemic heart diseases) [56]. ESWT is a treatment method that applies extracorporeal shock waves to lesions to aid revascularization and stimulate or reactivate the healing of bones and connective tissues such as tendons, thereby relieving pain and improving functions. Data suggest that in the field of tendinopathies ESWT can be considered not only as a symptomatologic therapy but rather a real curative treatment, able to relieve pain and inflammation in the short-medium term but also to positively interfere with tendon structure in a regenerative way [57]. In doing this, it causes changes in cells' metabolism and the permeability of endothelial cell tissues, leading to pain relief and having positive effects on soft tissues [58]. A recent systematic review demonstrated the effectiveness and safety of ESWT for frozen shoulder; ESWT determines the reduction of pain intensity, and it improves shoulder function, quality of life without adverse events [59].

6.2 Physiotherapy

Several studies have examined the effect of joint mobilization in patients with adhesive capsulitis, and although there is evidence that it may be beneficial, there is little evidence to support superior efficacy over other interventions [60–62].

Joint mobilization procedures are primarily directed to the glenohumeral joint to reduce pain and increase motion and function in patients with adhesive capsulitis. Mobilization techniques improve the normal extensibility of the shoulder capsule and stretch the tightened soft tissues to induce beneficial effects. Mulligan's mobilization-with-movement (MWM) treatment techniques, could be used. The most important points of the Mulligan Concept include the active participation of the patient and the elimination of pain during therapy [63]. A recent review of the literature analyzed 16 controlled clinical trial (CCT) or randomized controlled trial (RCT) studies that used MWMs demonstrating efficacy on pain and disability [64].

Also, stretching exercises appear to influence pain and improve ROM. The Harvard Special Health Report offers some stretching exercises that are effective in the treatment of adhesive capsulitis—pendulum stretch, towel stretch finger walk, cross-body reach, armpit stretch, starting to strengthen, outward rotation, inward rotation. These exercises can be performed with the physiotherapist or carried out as a home program [65].

No evidence exists to guide the optimal frequency, number of repetitions, or duration of stretching exercises. Stretching beyond painful limits may result in poorer outcomes. Therefore, stretching intensity that matches the given level of tissue irritability is indicated.

6.3 Manual myofascial therapy

Manual therapy may include myofascial work to release abnormal tension and restore mobility and function and identify fascial restrictions using motion testing and palpation.

In the myofascial treatment could be used simple techniques for muscle treatment and joint manipulations, such as:

- lateral elongation, a force applied with a right angle to the longitudinal axis of the muscle fascicles.

- linear extension and removal of the insertion points, with force applied proximally and distally to a dysfunctional area or muscle insertions, with longitudinal and parallel direction to the muscle fascicles.

- linear shortening and rapprochement of insertion points, with force applied proximally and distally to a dysfunctional area or muscle insertions, with longitudinal and parallel direction to the muscle fascicles.

- deep pressure, constant pressure on a zone of retraction or muscle tension or close to its bony insertion [66].

6.4 Minimally invasive treatments

6.4.1 Acupuncture

Acupuncture can be used to treat the pain of the frozen shoulder. It involves inserting needles into the skin at sites that vary from case to case and also depend on the practitioners' school of thought. Traditional Chinese medicine regarded acupuncture as an effective measure in aborting the signs and symptoms of frozen shoulder and in preventing future recurrence.

In the treatment of frozen shoulder, as in many other diseases, one in long, 30 gauge, disposable, sterilized, filiform needles are usually used. The sides of the application are defined as local points and distal points [67].

An integration approach can be ear acupuncture in the treatment of the frozen shoulder. According to traditional Chinese medicine, the sensitive spots on the auricle are anatomically and pathologically related to the affected shoulder joint [68] (**Figure 2**).

6.4.1.1 Kinesio taping (KT)

Kinesio taping is a complementary therapy based on the application of an elastic membrane that allows relieving pain. The effect on pain is pain modulation through pain gate control theory. The epidermis is equipped with a series of nerve receptors that, if subjected to a series of external stimuli, communicate with the underlying muscles. As a result, depending on how they are placed, the tapes can inhibit a contracted muscle or facilitate lymphatic flow, decreasing pain and inflammation [69]. The application KT

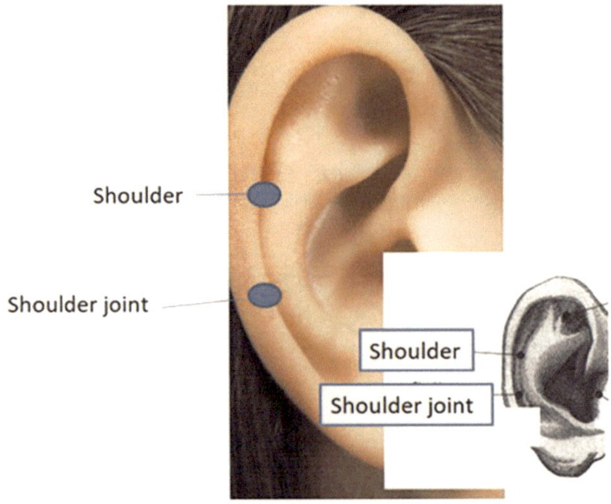

Figure 2.
Ear acupuncture in the treatment of frozen shoulder.

can produce local physiological changes that resulted in therapeutic effects, such as the relief of pain (pain gate mechanism, reducing muscle spasm) and improvement in ROM (tissue extensibility) [70, 71].

6.5 Operative treatments

6.5.1 Arthroscopic capsular release and manipulation under anesthetic (MUA)

Arthroscopic treatment is usually indicated in patients who do not respond to drug and/or rehabilitation therapy. Usually, during this procedure, a manipulation under anesthetic (MUA) is carried out as in this way, it is possible to reduce the potential damage by allowing it to be performed with less force. In addition to a general anesthetic, it is normal for a regional nerve block to be given. This causes postoperative numbness and enables the patient to get moving at the earliest possible stage. Intensive physiotherapy is regarded as essential to a good outcome.

6.6 Postural educational program

After a period of unconditioning typical of the acute phase of pain and contracture, it is necessary to learn again the correct body schema and achieve the complete recovery of postural control. It is possible through a progressive recovery of good motor control, thanks to the muscular selective reinforcement with the increasing development of strength in different patterns of movement, both the proprioceptive recovery. In the last rehabilitation phase it is necessary to restore the sensorimotor skills including proprioception static and dynamic balance either with aquatic rehabilitation therapy or through platform swing walkway, which is a common way to improve gait pattern through activation of sensory stimuli (visual, auditory, vestibular, and somatosensory) [72, 73].

0–2 weeks	Physical therapy Injection therapy Medication therapy Mobilization and manual therapy
2–4 weeks	Full passive range of motion should be achieved by 2–4 weeks Scapular and glenohumeral joint mobilization Begin rotator cuff retraining and strengthening, focus on restoring proper biomechanics
4–8 weeks	Progressive strength training contingent upon perfect biomechanics Development of independent home and gym program (aquatic microgravity environment)
8–10 weeks	Progression into normal activity and exercise program Long home maintenance program to include daily ROM exercises, rotator cuff program, and postural educational program

Table 3.
Summary of therapeutic strategies.

6.6.1 Summary of therapeutic strategies

See **Table 3**.

7. Conclusion

Often a rehabilitative success is defined by the return of normal motion rather than pain-free functional motion, but adhesive capsulitis is a challenging condition for both the physical therapist and patient. In fact, the healing process takes months to restore full mobility without pain, considering the presence of dense fibrotic tissue and the months of collagen remodeling required to recover soft tissue length. The rehabilitation of frozen shoulder is frequently prolonged despite multiple therapeutic methods because of the difficulty of acting on the degenerative process of the cartilage matrix and the progress of adhesive capsulitis. It is important to the diagnosis process and assessment to choose the best intervention or a combination of strategies for each patient. Although in scientific literature, a definition of the best rehabilitation approach is still needed, following an integrated, multifaceted, and combination of evidence-based approaches, therapeutic success can be achieved!

Disclosure

The author reports no conflicts of interest in this work.

Author details

Simona Maria Carmignano[1,2]

1 Department of Medicine, Surgery and Dentistry, "Salernitan Medical School", University of Salerno, Baronissi, Italy

2 C.T.R. Rehabilitation Therapeutic Center, Basilicata, Italy

*Address all correspondence to: simona.carmignano@gmail.com

References

[1] Neviaser JS. Adhesive capsulitis and the stiff and painful shoulder. The Orthopedic Clinics of North America. 1980;**11**:327-331

[2] Neviaser RJ. Painful conditions affecting the shoulder. Clinical Orthopaedics and Related Research. 1983:63-69

[3] Martin J, Kelley PT. Frozen shoulder: Evidence and a proposed model guiding rehabilitation. Journal of Orthopaedic & Sports Physical Therapy. 2009;**39**(2): 135-148

[4] Codman EA. The Shoulder: Rupture of the Supraspinatus Tendon and Other Lesions in or about the Subacromial Bursa. Boston, MA: T. Todd Co; 1934

[5] Neviaser JS. Adhesive capsulitis of the shoulder, a study of the pathological findings in periarthritis of the shoulder. The Journal of Bone & Joint Surgery. 1945;**27**:211-222

[6] Rangan A, Goodchild L, Gibson J, et al. Frozen shoulder [published correction appears in Shoulder Elbow. 2016;8(3):215]. Shoulder and Elbow. 2015;7(4):299-307. DOI: 10.1177/1758573215601779

[7] Hutchinson JW, Tierney GM, Parsons SL, Davis TR. Dupuytren's disease and frozen shoulder induced by treatment with a matrix metalloproteinase metalloproteinase inhibitor. Journal of Bone and Joint Surgery. British Volume (London). 1998; **80**:907-908

[8] Bunker TD, Reilly J, Baird KS, Hamblen DL. Expression of growth factors, cytokines and matrix metalloproteinases in frozen shoulder. Journal of Bone and Joint Surgery. 2000; **82**(5):768-773. DOI: 10.1302/0301-620X.82B5.9888

[9] Uhthoff HK, Boileau P. Primary frozen shoulder: Global capsular stiffness versus localized contracture. Clinical Orthopaedics and Related Research. 2007;**456**:79-84. DOI: 10.1097/BLO.0b013e318030846d

[10] Rodeo SA, Hannafin JA, Tom J, Warren RF, Wickiewicz TL. Immunolocalization of cytokines and their receptors in adhesive capsulitis of the shoulder. Journal of Orthopaedic Research. 1997;**15**(3):427-436. DOI: 10.1002/jor.1100150316

[11] Kilian O, Pfeil U, Wenisch S, Heiss C, Kraus R, Schnettler R. Enhanced alpha1(I) mRNA expression in frozen shoulder and dupuytren tissue. European Journal of Medical Research. 2007;**12**(12):585-590

[12] Bunker TD. Frozen shoulder: Unravelling the enigma. Annals of the Royal College of Surgeons of England. 1997;**79**(3):210-213

[13] Bunker TD, Anthony PP. The pathology of frozen shoulder. A dupuytren-like disease. Journal of Bone and Joint Surgery. 1995;**77**(5): 677-683

[14] Cho CH, Song KS, Kim BS, Kim DH, Lho YM. Biological aspect of pathophysiology for frozen shoulder. BioMed Research International. 2018; **2018**:7274517. Published 2018. DOI: 10.1155/2018/7274517

[15] Hand GCR, Athanasou NA, Matthews T, Carr AJ. The pathology of frozen shoulder. Journal of Bone and Joint Surgery. 2007;**89**(7):928-932. DOI: 10.1302/0301-620X.89B7.19097

[16] Kanbe K, Inoue K, Inoue Y, Chen Q. Inducement of mitogen-activated protein kinases in frozen shoulders. Journal of Orthopaedic Science. 2009; **14**(1):56-61. DOI: 10.1007/s00776-008-1295-6

[17] Cadogan A, Mohammed KD. Shoulder pain in primary care: Frozen shoulder. Journal of Primary Health Care. 2016;**8**(1):44-51. DOI: 10.1071/HC15018

[18] Jason E, Okechukwu A, Anakwenze William J, Joseph W, Abboud A. Current review of adhesive capsulitis. Journal of Shoulder and Elbow Surgery. 2011;**20**: 502-514

[19] Neviaser RJ, Neviaser TJ. The frozen shoulder. Diagnosis and management. Clinical Orthopaedics and Related Research. 1987:59-64

[20] Vermeulen HM, Obermann WR, Burger BJ, et al. End-range mobilization techniques in adhesive capsulitis of the shoulder joint: A multiple-subject case report. Physical Therapy. 2000;**80**: 1204-1213

[21] Armstrong A. Diagnosis and clinical assessment of a stiff shoulder. Shoulder and Elbow. 2015;**7**(2):128-134. DOI: 10.1177/1758573215569340

[22] Kessler RM. The shoulder. In: Kessler RM, Hertling D, editors. Management of Common Musculoskeletal Disorders. Philadelphia: Harper & Row; 1983. pp. 274-310

[23] Padua R, Padua L, Ceccarelli E, et al. Italian version of the disability of the arm, shoulder and hand (dash) questionnaire. Cross-cultural adaptation and validation. The Journal of Hand Surgery. 2003;**28**(2): 179-186. DOI: 10.1016/S0266-7681(02) 00303-0

[24] Richards RR, An KN, Bigliani LU, Friedman RJ, Gartsman GM, Gristina AG, et al. A standardized method for the assessment of shoulder function. Journal of Shoulder and Elbow Surgery. 1994; **3**(6):347-352

[25] Williams JW, Holleman DR, Simel DL. Measuring shoulder function with the shoulder pain and disability index. The Journal of Rheumatology. 1995; **22**(4):727-732

[26] Hershkovich O, Shapira S, Sela Y, Botser I. Role of radiographs in shoulder pathology: A clinical review. Reports in Medical Imaging. 2014;7:75-80. DOI: 10.2147/RMI.S35587

[27] Tandon A, Dewan S, Bhatt S, Jain AK, Kumari R. Sonography in diagnosis of adhesive capsulitis of the shoulder: A case-control study. Journal of Ultrasound. 2017;**20**(3):227-236. Published 2017. DOI: 10.1007/s40477-017-0262-5

[28] Do JG, Hwang JT, Yoon KJ, Lee YT. Correlation of ultrasound findings with clinical stages and impairment in adhesive capsulitis of the shoulder. Orthopaedic Journal of Sports Medicine. 2021;**9**(5):23259671211003675. DOI: 10.1177/23259671211003675

[29] Cheng X, Zhang Z, Xuanyan G, Li T, Li J, Yin L, et al. Adhesive capsulitis of the shoulder: Evaluation with US-arthrography using a sonographic contrast agent. Scientific Reports. 2017; **7**(1):5551

[30] Homsi C, Bordalo-Rodrigues M, da Silva JJ, Stump XM. Ultrasound in adhesive capsulitis of the shoulder: Is assessment of the coracohumeral ligament a valuable diagnostic tool? Skeletal Radiology. 2006;**35**(9): 673-678

[31] Wu CH, Chen WS, Wang TG. Elasticity of the coracohumeral ligament in patients with adhesive capsulitis of the shoulder. Radiology. 2016;**278**(2): 458-464

[32] Michelin P, Delarue Y, Duparc F, Dacher JN. Thickening of the inferior glenohumeral capsule: An ultrasound sign for shoulder capsular contracture. European Radiology. 2013;**23**(10): 2802-2806

[33] Lee JC, Sykes C, Saifuddin A, Connell D. Adhesive capsulitis: Sonographic changes in the rotator cuff interval with arthroscopic correlation. Skeletal Radiology. 2005;**34**(9):522-527

[34] Sofka CM, Ciavarra GA, Hannafin JA, Cordasco FA, Potter HG. Magnetic resonance imaging of adhesive capsulitis: Correlation with clinical staging. HSS Journal. 2008;**4**(2):164-169. DOI: 10.1007/s11420-008-9088-1

[35] Loyd JA, Loyd HM. Adhesive capsulitis of the shoulder: Arthrographic diagnosis and treatment. Southern Medical Journal. 1983;**76**(7):879-883

[36] Neviaser AS, Hannafin JA. Adhesive capsulitis: A review of current treatment. The American Journal of Sports Medicine. 2010;**38**:2346-2356

[37] Uppal HS, Evans JP, Smith C. Frozen shoulder: A systematic review of therapeutic options. World Journal of Orthopedics. 2015;**18**:263-268

[38] Melzer C, Hoffmann S, Wallny T, et al. Frozen shoulder—Treatment and results. Archives of Orthopaedic and Traumatic Surgery. 1995;**114**:87-91. DOI: 10.1007/BF00422832

[39] Ryans I, Montgomery A, Galway R, Kernohan W, G. McKane R. A randomized controlled trial of intra-articular triamcinolone and/or physiotherapy in shoulder capsulitis. Rheumatology. 2005;**44**:529-535

[40] Dacre JE, Beeney N, Scott DL. Injections and physiotherapy for the painful stiff shoulder. Annals of the Rheumatic Diseases. 1989;**48**:322-325

[41] Blanchard V, Barr S, Cerisola FL. The effectiveness of corticosteroid injections compared with physiotherapeutic interventions for adhesive capsulitis: A systematic review. Physiotherapy. 2010;**6**:95-107

[42] Harris JD, Griesser MJ, Copelan A, Jones GL. Treatment of adhesive capsulitis with intra-articular hyaluronate: A systematic review. International Journal of Shoulder Surgery. 2011;**5**(2):31-37. DOI: 10.4103/0973-6042.83194

[43] Abate M, Schiavone C, Salini V. The use of hyaluronic acid after tendon surgery and in tendinopathies. BioMed Research International. 2014;**2014**: 783632. DOI: 10.1155/2014/783632

[44] Wright A, Sluka KA. Nonpharmacological treatments for musculoskeletal pain. The Clinical Journal of Pain. 2001;**17**(1):33-46

[45] Robertson VJ, Baker KG. A review of therapeutic ultrasound - effectiveness studies. Physical Therapy. 2001;**81**(7): 1339-1350

[46] Basford JR. Therapeutic physical agents. In: De Lisa JA, editor. Physical Medicine and Rehabilitation. Principles and Practice. Philadelphia: Lippincott Williams & Wilkins; 2005. p. 251e70

[47] Saggini R, Di Stefano A, Carmignano SM, Ancona E, Di Felice PA, Bellomo RG. The Treatment with Low Frequency Acoustic Pressure Waves (Ultrasound

Diathermy): Therapeutic Considerations and Clinical Reports. University Centre of Physical and Rehabilitation Medicine, Chair of Physical and Rehabilitation Medicine, University "G. d'Annunzio" – Chieti. Available from: https://www.researchgate.net/publication/322065721_

[48] Bellomo RG, Carmignano S, Saggini R. The applied mechanical vibration as ultrasound energy. In: Saggini R, editor. The Mechanical Vibration: Therapeutic Effects and Applications. Sharjah, United Arab Emirates: Bentham Science Publishers; 2017. pp. 89-180 (92)

[49] Philadelphia Panel. Philadelphia panel evidence-based clinical practice guidelines on selected rehabilitation interventions for shoulder pain. In: Database of Abstracts of Reviews of Effects (DARE): Quality-Assessed Reviews [Internet]. York (UK): Centre for Reviews and Dissemination (UK); 2001. Available from: https://www.ncbi.nlm.nih.gov/books/NBK68663/

[50] Dogru H, Basaran S, Sarpel T. Effectiveness of therapeutic ultrasound in adhesive capsulitis. Joint, Bone, Spine. 2008;**75**:445-450. DOI: 10.1016/j.jbspin.2007.07.016

[51] Ebadi S, Forogh B, Fallah E, Ghazani AB. Does ultrasound therapy add to the effects of exercise and mobilization in frozen shoulder? A pilot randomized double-blind clinical trial. Journal of Bodywork and Movement Therapies. 2017;**21**:781-787

[52] Doner G, Guven Z, Atalay A, Celiker R. Evaluation of mulligan's technique for adhesive capsulitis of the shoulder. Journal of Rehabilitation Medicine. 2013; **45**:87-91

[53] Paolucci T, Pezzi L, Centra AM, Giannandrea N, Bellomo RG, Saggini R. Electromagnetic field therapy: A rehabilitative perspective in the management of musculoskeletal pain—A systematic review. Journal of Pain Research. 2020;**13**:1385-1400. DOI: 10.2147/JPR.S231778

[54] Quittan M, Schuhfried O, Wiesinger GF, Fialka-Moser V. Clinical effectiveness of magnetic field therapy—A review of the literature. Acta Medica Austriaca. 2000;**27**(3):61-68

[55] Iwasa K, Reddi AH. Pulsed electromagnetic fields and tissue engineering of the joints. Tissue Engineering. Part B, Reviews. 2018; **24**(2):144-154

[56] D'Agostino MC, Carmignano SM, Saggini A. The applied mechanical vibration as extracorporeal shock wave. In: Saggini R, editor. The Mechanical Vibration: Therapeutic Effects and Applications. Sharjah, United Arab Emirates: Bentham Science Publishers; 2017. pp. 181-219 (39)

[57] Agostino MCD, Frairia R, Romeo P, Amelio E, Berta L, Bosco V, et al. Extracorporeal shockwaves as regenerative therapy in orthopedic traumatology: A narrative review from basic research to clinical practice. Journal of Biological Regulators and Homeostatic Agents. 2016;**30**(2):323-332

[58] Park C, Lee S, Yi CW, Lee K. The effects of extracorporeal shock wave therapy on frozen shoulder patients' pain and functions. Journal of Physical Therapy Science. 2015;**27**(12):3659-3661. DOI: 10.1589/jpts.27.3659

[59] Dong-zi C, Wang C, Qing Z, Liu L. Effectiveness of extracorporeal shock-wave therapy for frozen shoulder. Medicine. 2019;**98**(7):e14506. DOI: 10.1097/MD.0000000000014506

[60] Johnson AJ, Godges JJ, Zimmerman GJ, Ounanian LL. The effect of anterior versus posterior glide joint mobilization on external rotation range of motion in patients with shoulder adhesive capsulitis. Journal of Orthopaedic & Sports Physical Therap. 2007;**37**:88-99. DOI: 10.2519/jospt.2007.2307

[61] Nicholson GG et al. The Journal of Orthopaedic and Sports Physical Therapy. 1985;**6**:238-246. BMJ. 1998;317: 1292-1296

[62] Vermeulen HM, Rozing PM, Obermann WR, le Cessie S, Vliet Vlieland TP. Comparison of high-grade and low-grade mobilization techniques in the management of adhesive capsulitis of the shoulder: Randomizedcontrolled trial. Physical Therapy. 2006;**86**:355-368

[63] Hing W, Hall T, Rivett D, Vicenzino B, Mulligan B. The Mulligan Concept of Manual Therapy-eBook: Textbook of Techniques. Elsevier Health Sciences; 2014

[64] Stathopoulos N, Dimitriadis Z, Koumantakis GA. Effectiveness of Mulligan's mobilization with movement techniques on pain and disability of peripheral joints: A systematic review with meta-analysis between 2008-2017. Physiotherapy. 2019;**105**(1):1-9. DOI: 10.1016/j.physio.2018.10.001. Epub 2018. Erratum in: Physiotherapy. 2020;106:219

[65] Elson L, Gardiner J. For more exercises to improve your balance and prevent falls, increase your flexibility, and even help relieve arthritis, back, and knee pain, buy the Harvard Special Health Report Stretching: 35 exercises to improve flexibility and reduce pain

[66] Yang JL, Chang CW, Chen SY, Wang SF, Lin JJ. Mobilization techniques in subjects with frozen shoulder syndrome: Randomized multiple-treatment trial. Physical Therapy. 2007; **87**:1307-1315

[67] Tukmachi ES. Frozen shoulder: A comparison of Western and traditional Chinese approaches and a clinical study of its acupuncture treatment. Acupuncture in Medicine. 1999;**17**(1): 9-21. DOI: 10.1136/aim.17.1.9

[68] Liu Z editor. Essentials of Chinese Acupuncture. Beijing: Academy of Traditional Chinese Medicine. Springer-Verlag London; 2009. doi: 10.1007/ 978-1-84882-593-2

[69] Panchbudhe SA, Praveen Kumar Y, Choudhary S, Chiwhane A. Role of the physiotherapist to promote physical activity in physical therapy settings: A questionnaire study. International Journal of Current Research and Review. 2020;**12**(14 Special Issue): 50-55

[70] Deshmukh N, Kahile M, Chaudhary N, Panchbhudhe S, Gawande V. Adjunct effect of kinesiotaping on adhesive capsulities of shoulder joint. International Journal of Current Research and Review. 2021; **13**(08):48-53. DOI: 10.31782/ IJCRR.2021.13818

[71] Hanchard NC, Goodchild L, Thompson J, O'Brien T, Davison D, Richardson C. Evidence-based clinical guidelines for the diagnosis, assessment and physiotherapy management of contracted (frozen) shoulder: Quick reference summary. Physiotherapy. 2012;**98**(2):117-120. DOI: 10.1016/ j.physio.2012.01.001

[72] Stupay K, Neviaser A. Management of adhesive capsulitis. Orthopedic Research and Reviews. 2015;7:83-94. DOI: 10.2147/ORR.S56317

[73] Saggini R, Bellomo RG, Carmignano SM, Saggini A. Cancer pain—The role of an integrated, comprehensive rehabilitation program in its management. In: Leticia R, Silva IV, editors. Updates on Cancer Treatment. Rijeka: Edit IntechOpen; 2015. DOI: 10.5772/60548

Section 2

Rotator Cuff Arthropathy

Chapter 4

Subacromial InSpace Balloon Interposition for Massive Irreparable Rotator Cuff Tears

Vladimir Senekovic

Abstract

Massive rotator cuff tears are a challenging problem for treatment. The best results we can still achieve with reconstruction. For treatment of massive rotator cuff tears when reconstruction is not possible, a new method has been developed recently: the implantation of the biodegradable balloon spacer/InSpace™ balloon/filled with the saline in the subacromial space. The main characteristic of this method is that to allow gliding of the humeral head against acromion without friction and to depress the humeral head for 2–3 mm. This depression is just enough that the humerus is in a better center of rotation that allows the deltoid muscle more strength—better vector forces for the deltoid muscle. This function of the balloon permits better deltoid activation and compensation through the arc of motion. Results of our first study and results of others show clinical safety and efficacy of the insertion of the InSpace™ balloon in a group of patients with massive irreparable rotator cuff tears. The insertion of this device shows significantly better early improvement, significant improvement in subjective pain scores, and a decrease in reported night pain. The measurement of the Total Constant score showed statistically significant improvement after insertion of the InSpace™ balloon at 5 years of follow-up. Generally, all studies show 75–80% of good results.

Keywords: massive rotator cuff tear, subacromial balloon spacer

1. Introduction

- The deployment of an inflatable resorbable balloon into the subacromial space is indicated in patients with massive-irreparable rotator cuff tears [1–15].

- Rotator cuff tears (RCTs) are among the commonest tendon injuries seen in orthopedic patients resulting in significant pain and disability [16–22].

- Irreparable RCTs are those where the rupture at least two tendons is present, tendons are retracted, atrophy of muscles and bigger degree of fatty degeneration are present [4, 23].

- In these situations, direct repair refixation of the tendon at the point of insertion is usually not possible despite extensive soft-tissue mobilization and release [24–27].
- The InSpace ™ system is a biodegradable balloon that is made for arthroscopic insertion into the subacromial space following bursa excision. The pre-shaped balloon is produced from a copolymer of poly-L-lactide-co-ε-caprolactone in a 70: 30 ratio, which biodegrades over a period of 12 months. The insertion of this balloon into the subacromial space is a low-risk procedure [6–9]. The aim of this is mainly to allow gliding of the humeral head against acromion without friction and to depress the humeral head for 2–3 mm. This depression is just enough that the humerus is in a better center of rotation that allows the deltoid muscle more strength—better vector forces for the deltoid muscle. This function of the balloon permits better deltoid activation and compensation through the arc of motion (**Figure 1**) [10].
- We have to be aware not to put the balloon into osteoarthritic joint—as such a joint balloon is not really effective [6, 8].

2. Preoperative assessment

2.1 Clinical assessment

- Patients describe chronicity of the difficulties: chronic night pain, pain at motion, limited range of motion [28, 29].
- Examination assesses the location of pain [4, 13].

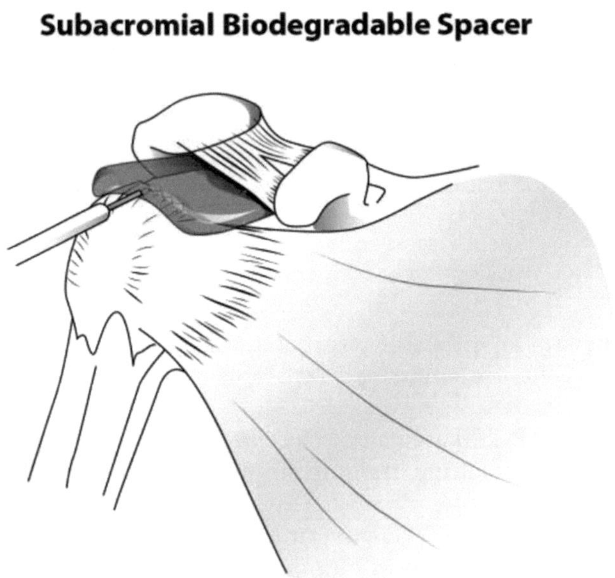

Figure 1.
Schematic representation of the InSpace ™ balloon deployment and inflation in the subacromial space.

- Pain can limit the range of motion. The range of motion is usually limited under 90° of anteflexion and abduction [13].
- Muscle strength is usually diminished [4, 23].
- Atrophy of the m. supraspinatus and m. infraspinatus is usually visible [23].

2.2 Imaging assessment

2.2.1 Radiographs

- Anteroposterior and lateral views detect possible superior migration of the humeral head and osteoarthritic joint [23].

2.2.2 Ultra sound (US)

- US is useful for detecting the tear and size of the tear.
- We can see calcium depots and muscle atrophy [23].

2.2.3 Multi resonance imaging (MRI) arthrography

- MRI arthrography is nearly 100° accurate to show RC tear and size of the tear.
- We can determine tendon retraction.
- We can determine atrophy of the muscle and degree of fatty degeneration.
- We can detect osteoarthritic changes in the joint [4, 23].

3. Timing for surgery

- The mean duration of symptoms because of the RCT prior to surgery has to be at least 3 months at patients over 60 years of age with documented failure of conservative treatment. All younger, we operate earlier [7, 21, 23].
- At operation we always try to mobilize the cuff and make reconstruction or partial reconstruction. If this is not possible, then we decide on the implantation of the balloon [5].

4. Surgical preparation

4.1 Surgical equipment

- Complete arthroscopic set with a shaver and a high-frequency electrode.
- An arthroscopic pump.

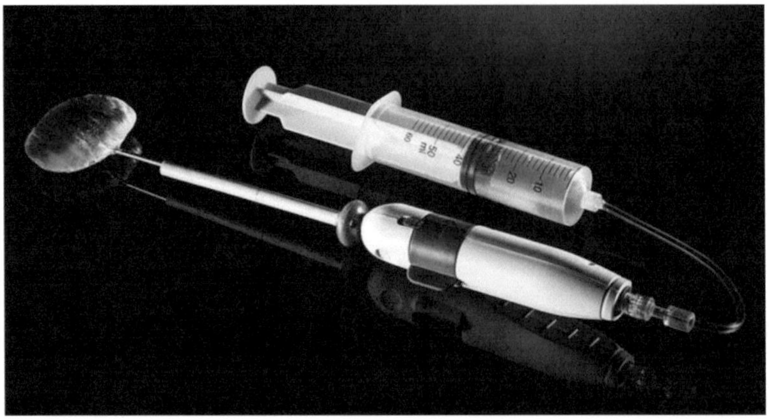

Figure 2.
InSpaceTM resorbable balloon—The ballon has been inflated already.

- Entire arthroscopic RC repair set includes anchor sutures or/and arthroscopic tunnel device.
- InSpaceTM resorbable balloons of three dimensions (**Figure 2**) with appropriate 20 ml syringe [6].

4.2 Equipment positioning

- The arthroscopic monitor faces the surgeon on the opposite side of the table at the level of the patient's shoulder [2, 7].

4.3 Patient positioning

- We have to put the patient in the beach chair position or in lateral decubitus position with the arm in a special holder like at all other shoulder arthroscopic procedures. For the lateral decubitus position, we need a special holding device for the body of the patient [2, 7].

4.4 Further preparation

- Implantation of the material justify antibiotic prophylaxis [2, 7].

5. Surgical technique

- We perform all shoulder operations with the patient in a beach-chair position.
- Nowadays, we perform shoulder arthroscopic procedures mainly in regional anesthesia (scalene block). In only a few cases, we perform in general anesthesia [6, 7].
- We use three standard arthroscopic ports (anterior, lateral, posterior, or posterolateral).

- At surgery we remove first partially the subacromial bursa (**Figure 3**), then we debride the tear and release the tendon. After this, we try to draw the edge of the tendons with an arthroscopic clamp to the footprint region (**Figure 4**). A decision is made to insert the balloon when it is obvious that the RCT is irreparable [6, 7, 30].

- We usually perform tenotomy of the tendon of the long head of m. biceps brachii. But this is not necessary [28, 31].

- Measurement of the distance between the lateral border of the acromion and the superior rim of the glenoid and defining the extent of any tear extension (**Figure 5**) [17].

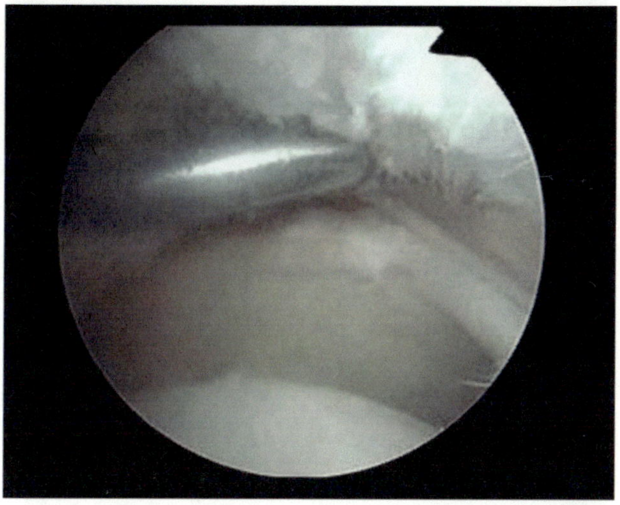

Figure 3.
Debridement of the subacromial space.

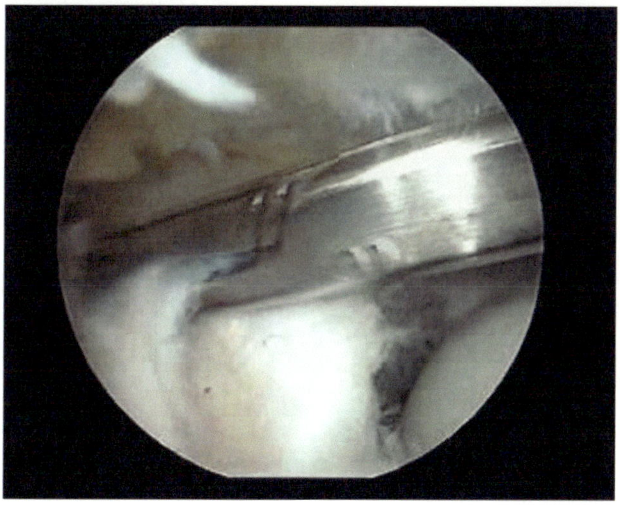

Figure 4.
Grasping the edges of the tendons with an arthroscopic clamp in an attempt to draw it to the footprint region.

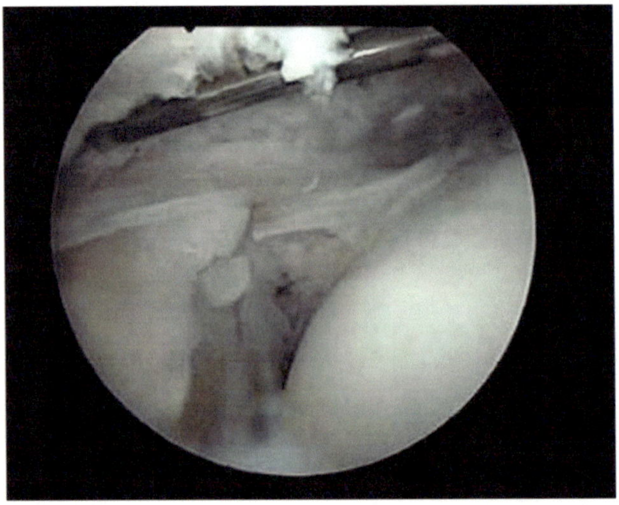

Figure 5.
Measurement of the distance between the lateral border of the acromion and the superior rim of the glenoid.

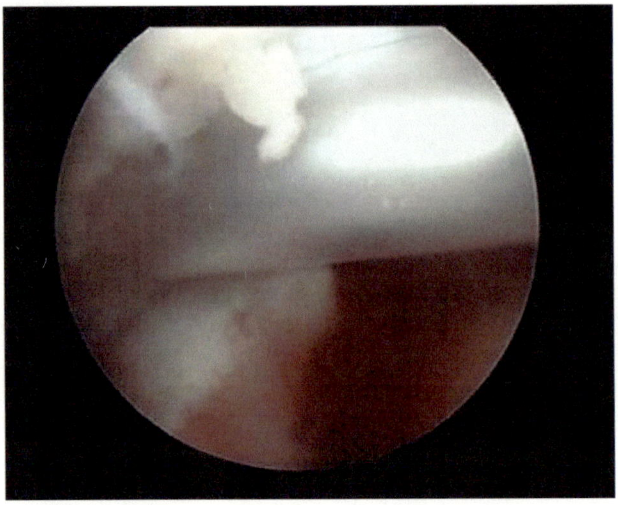

Figure 6.
Insertion of the proper balloon (cylindrical shape, insertion tube is removed from the joint).

- Then we choose the balloon size (small, medium or large) according to measurements.

- Insertion of the proper balloon is aided by folding it into a cylindrical shape inside an insertion tube (**Figure 6**).

- Once positioned in the subacromial space, the balloon is inflated with saline permitting frictionless gliding of the humeral head against the acromion. For each size we have to fill with the proper amount of the saline—it is written on the package (**Figures** 7 and **8**) [6, 7].

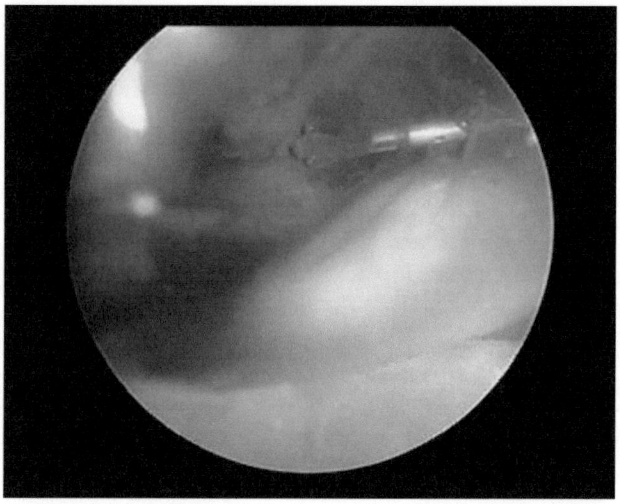

Figure 7.
Inflation of the balloon in the subacromial space.

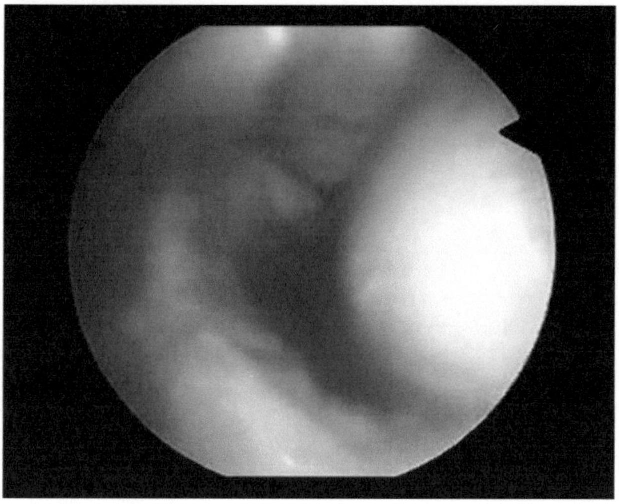

Figure 8.
Balloon is inflated in the subacromial space, we can see that humeral head is pushed down.

- Then we simply turn around the green ring on the handle holder and cut of insertion device from the balloon.

- After this we can move the arm and suture the ports.

6. Postoperative course

6.1 Postoperative regime

- Medications: pain killer, nonsteroidal anti-inflammatory drugs (NSAI).

- 5–7 days of immobilization of the arm during walking with broad arm sling.
- Immediate mobilization without limitations.
- Further physiotherapy.
- Outpatient visit at day 7 and 21 to check movement [6, 7].

6.2 Early phase postoperative complications

- Swelling of the shoulder
- There may be an obvious swelling in the arm caused by the contracted biceps muscle (**"Popeye sign"**)—this sometimes develops due to tenotomy of the long head of the biceps brachii muscle [28, 31].

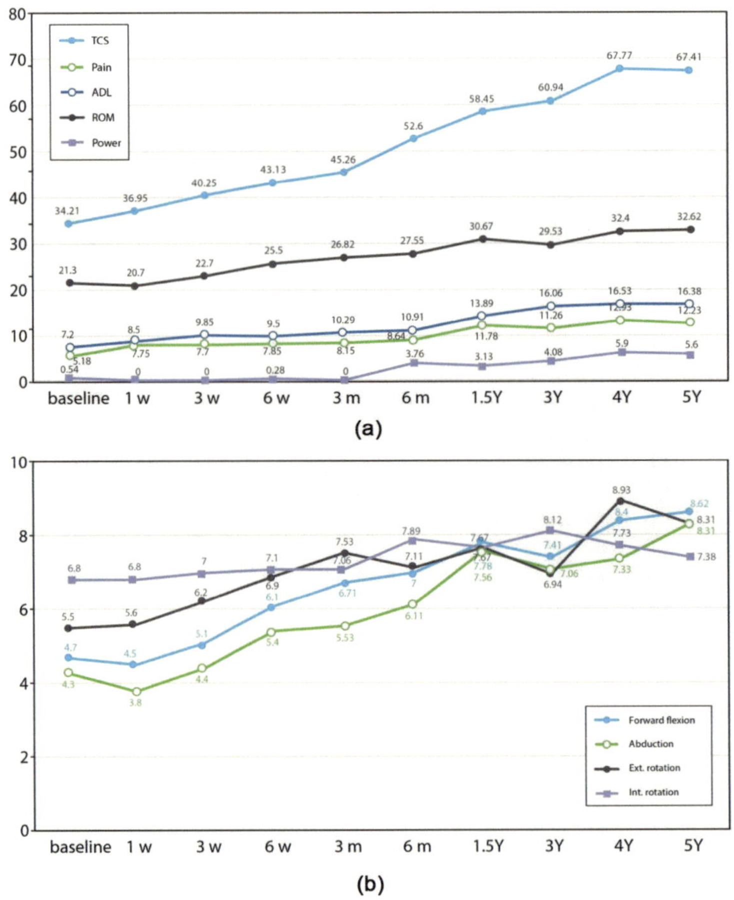

Figure 9.
(a) graphical presentation of constant variables following biodegradable spacer insertion. TCS—total constant score, pain score, ADL—Activity of daily living, ROM—Range of motion, power. Figure presents change in score from baseline to 5 years following insertion. Values are presented as means ±SD. (b)-graphical presentation of range of motion scores variables during 5 years follow-up. Active, pain-free range of elevation: 2 points per 30°; 0 = worst, 10 = best; position of hand:0 = worst, 10 = best. Values are presented as means.

7. Conclusion

- Our first study and results of other studies show clinical safety and efficacy of the insertion of the InSpace™ balloon in a group of patients with massive irreparable rotator cuff tears [6, 7].
- The insertion of this device shows significantly better early improvement, significant improvement in subjective pain scores, and a decrease in reported night pain. The measurement of the Total Constant score showed statistically significant improvement after insertion of the InSpace™ balloon at 5 years of follow-up. Generally, all studies show 75–80% of good results. (**Figure 9**) [6, 11–13].

Author details

Vladimir Senekovic
Arbormea Medical, Ljubljana, Slovenia

*Address all correspondence to: vladimir.senekovic@arbormea.com

References

[1] Green A. Chronic massive rotator cuff tears: evaluation and management. The Journal of the American Academy of Orthopaedic Surgeons. 2003;**11**(5):321-331

[2] Gerber C, Wirth SH, Farshad M. Treatment options for massive rotator cuff tears. Journal of Shoulder and Elbow Surgery. 2011;**20**(2 Suppl):S20-S29

[3] Anley CM, Chan SK, Snow M. Arthroscopic treatment options for irreparable rotator cuff tears of the shoulder. World Journal of Orthopedics. 2014;**5**(5):557-565

[4] Burkhart SS, JRH B, Richards DP, Zlatkin MB, Larsen M. Arthroscopic repair of massive rotator cuff tears with stage 3 and 4 fatty degeneration. Arthroscopy: Journal of Arthroscopic Related Surgery. 2007;**23**(4):347-354

[5] Berth A, Neumann W, Awiszus F, Pap G. Massive rotator cuff tears: functional outcome after debridement or arthroscopic partial repair. Journal of Orthopaedics and Traumatology. 2010;**11**(1):13-20

[6] Senekovic V, Poberaj B, Kovacic L, Mikek M, Adar E, Dekel A. Prospective clinical study of a novel biodegradable sub-acromial spacer in treatment of massive irreparable rotator cuff tears. European Journal of Orthopaedic Surgery and Traumatology. 2013;**23**(3):311-316

[7] Savarese E, Romeo R. New solution for massive, irreparable rotator cuff tears: the subacromial "biodegradable spacer." Arthroscopy Techniques. 2012;**1**(1):e69-e74

[8] Kilinc AS, Ebrahimzadeh MH, Lafosse L. Subacromial internal spacer for rotator cuff tendon repair: "the balloon technique." Arthroscopy Journal of Arthroscopic Related Surgery. 2009;**25**(8):921-924

[9] Sartoretti C, Sartoretti-Schefer S, Duff C, Buchmann P. Angioplasty balloon catheters used for distraction of the ankle joint. Arthroscopy: The Journal of Arthroscopic & Related Surgery. 1996;**12**(1):82-86

[10] Chaudhury S, Holland C, Thompson MS, Vollrath F, Carr AJ. Tensile and shear mechanical properties of rotator cuff repair patches. Journal of Shoulder and Elbow Surgery. 2012;**21**(9):1168-1176

[11] Kukkonen J, Kauko T, Vahlberg T, Joukainen A, Äärimaa V. Investigating minimal clinically important difference for Constant score in patients undergoing rotator cuff surgery. Journal of Shoulder and Elbow Surgery. 2013;**22**(12):1650-1655

[12] Conboy VB, Morris RW, Kiss J, Carr AJ. An evaluation of the Constant-Murley shoulder assessment. Journal of Bone and Joint Surgery. British Volume (London). 1996;**78**(2):229-232

[13] Constant CR, Murley AH. A clinical method of functional assessment of the shoulder. Clinical Orthopaedics. 1987;**214**:160-164

[14] Katolik LI, Romeo AA, Cole BJ, Verma NN, Hayden JK, Bach BR. Normalization of the Constant score. Journal of Shoulder and Elbow Surgery. 2005;**14**(3):279-285

[15] Gustavson K, von Soest T, Karevold E, Røysamb E. Attrition and generalizability in longitudinal studies:

findings from a 15-year population-based study and a Monte Carlo simulation study. BMC Public Health. 2012;**12**:918

[16] Omid R, Lee B. Tendon transfers for irreparable rotator cuff tears. The Journal of the American Academy of Orthopaedic Surgeons. 2013;**21**(8):492-501

[17] Warner JJ. Management of massive irreparable rotator cuff tears: the role of tendon transfer. Instructional Course Lectures. 2001;**50**:63-71

[18] Hirooka A, Yoneda M, Wakaitani S, Isaka Y, Hayashida K, Fukushima S, et al. Augmentation with a Gore-Tex patch for repair of large rotator cuff tears that cannot be sutured. Journal of Orthopaedic Science. 2002;**7**(4):451-456

[19] Moore DR, Cain EL, Schwartz ML, Clancy WG. Allograft reconstruction for massive, irreparable rotator cuff tears. The American Journal of Sports Medicine. 2006;**34**(3):392-396

[20] Ozaki J, Fujimoto S, Masuhara K, Tamai S, Yoshimoto S. Reconstruction of chronic massive rotator cuff tears with synthetic materials. Clinical Orthopaedics. 1986;**202**:173-183

[21] Hawkins RJ, Misamore GW, Hobeika PE. Surgery for full-thickness rotator-cuff tears. The Journal of Bone and Joint Surgery. American Volume. 1985;**67**(9):1349-1355

[22] Rockwood CA, Williams GR, Burkhead WZ. Débridement of degenerative, irreparable lesions of the rotator cuff. The Journal of Bone and Joint Surgery. American Volume. 1995;**77**(6):857-866

[23] Goutallier D, Postel JM, Bernageau J, Lavau L, Voisin MC. Fatty muscle degeneration in cuff ruptures. Pre- and postoperative evaluation by CT scan. Clinical Orthopaedics. 1994;**304**:78-83

[24] Gerber C. Latissimus dorsi transfer for the treatment of irreparable tears of the rotator cuff. Clinical Orthopaedics. 1992;**275**:152-160

[25] Scheibel M, Lichtenberg S, Habermeyer P. Reversed arthroscopic subacromial decompression for massive rotator cuff tears. Journal of Shoulder and Elbow Surgery. 2004;**13**(3):272-278

[26] Nové-Josserand L, Costa P, Liotard J-P, Safar J-F, Walch G, Zilber S. Results of latissimus dorsi tendon transfer for irreparable cuff tears. Orthopaedics & Traumatology: Surgery & Research. 2009;**95**(2):108-113

[27] Lee BG, Cho NS, Rhee YG. Results of arthroscopic decompression and tuberoplasty for irreparable massive rotator cuff tears. Arthroscopy: The Journal of Arthroscopic & Related Surgery. 2011;**27**(10):1341-1350

[28] Walch G, Edwards TB, Boulahia A, Nové-Josserand L, Neyton L, Szabo I. Arthroscopic tenotomy of the long head of the biceps in the treatment of rotator cuff tears: clinical and radiographic results of 307 cases. Journal of Shoulder and Elbow Surgery. 2005;**14**(3):238-246

[29] Wong I, Burns J, Snyder S. Arthroscopic GraftJacket repair of rotator cuff tears. Journal of Shoulder and Elbow Surgery. 2010;**19**(2 Suppl):104-109

[30] Gartsman GM. Arthroscopic acromioplasty for lesions of the rotator cuff. The Journal of Bone and Joint Surgery. American Volume. 1990;**72**(2):169-180

[31] Szabó I, Boileau P, Walch G. The proximal biceps as a pain generator and results of tenotomy. Sports Medicine and Arthroscopy Review. 2008;**16**(3):180-186

Chapter 5

Outpatient Total Shoulder Replacement Procedures

Brandon J. Erickson, Yousef Shishani and Reuben Gobezie

Abstract

The number of total shoulder arthroplasty (TSA) and reverse total shoulder arthroplasty (RTSA) procedures performed each year has continued to rise. While these procedures were historically done in the inpatient setting, many surgeons have migrated to performing TSA and RTSA in the outpatient setting. This can either involve sending patients home the same day from the hospital or performing these in an outpatient center. Specific protocols should be followed in regard to patient selection to minimize the risk of complications and readmission. Similarly, a team approach between the anesthesiologist and the surgeon is critical to ensure adequate pain control. Use of tranexamic acid (TXA), a preoperative nerve block as well as specific combinations of preoperative and postoperative medications are helpful in creating an optimal environment in which to perform the shoulder arthroplasty for the patient. When done well, TSA and RTSA can successfully be performed as an outpatient with a very high success rate and a low risk of complications.

Keywords: total shoulder arthroplasty (TSA), reverse total shoulder arthroplasty (RTSA), outpatient, hospital, surgical center, shoulder, arthroplasty, ambulatory, complication, readmission, outcome

1. Introduction

The number of total shoulder arthroplasty (TSA) and reverse total shoulder arthroplasty (RTSA) procedures performed each year has continued to rise, and will continue to rise as the population ages and lives longer (**Figure 1**) [1–3]. While shoulder arthroplasty has historically been performed in the inpatient setting, over the several years, many surgeons have moved to performing TSA/RTSA in the outpatient setting. Performing shoulder arthroplasty in the outpatient setting decreases cost to the healthcare system as well as provides an excellent patient experience. Recent studies have shown excellent results with few complications in patients who have undergone outpatient TSA/RTSA [4–7]. However, not every patient is a candidate for an outpatient shoulder arthroplasty.

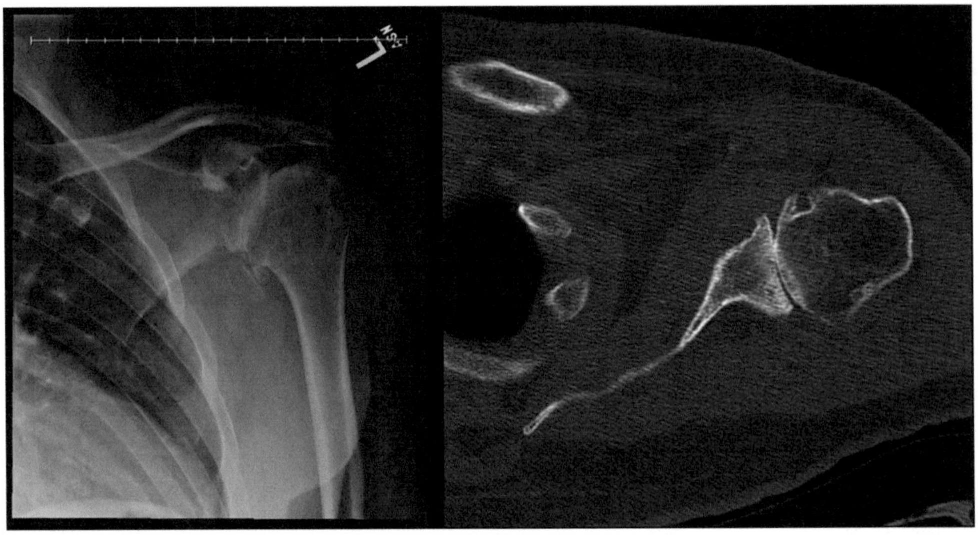

Figure 1.
Examples of advanced arthritis (Coronal X-ray and axial CT scan).

2. What patients are eligible for outpatient shoulder arthroplasty?

While a great many patients are candidates for TSA and RTSA, not every patient is a candidate for a shoulder arthroplasty in an outpatient setting. First, some patients may not be comfortable having surgery in an outpatient center and some insurance companies may not be accepted by the outpatient center. In these cases the surgery should be done in the hospital setting. It also helps if patients have a good home support system to help them with activities of daily living following surgery. While they will be able to do many things on their own, there will be some things that they will likely need help with. There are many services an outpatient center does not have that a hospital has, so patients at increased risk for complications, bleeding, breathing issues, etc. should not have their shoulder arthroplasty done in an outpatient center. The authors have developed criteria to determine whether patients are good candidates for shoulder arthroplasty in the outpatient setting.

From a medical perspective, patients who are American Society of Anesthesiology (ASA) 1 and 2 are often eligible. Occasionally patients who are ASA 3 are eligible, but this should be a case-by-case decision. Patients under 65 years of age are often better suited for an outpatient arthroplasty, although older, high functioning patients can be good candidates as well. Patients should be off chronic narcotics before having an outpatient shoulder arthroplasty and must be willing to participate in a multimodal pain management program. Furthermore, the patient should be a good candidate for a regional block for pain control. The following is a list of relative contraindications to patients having their TSA/RTSA in an outpatient setting. Any patients who have conditions on this list may require a proper medical/cardiology and anesthesia evaluation preoperatively.

- Cardiac
  - Significant heart disease
    - Poor LVEF (<50%)

        - Ischemic heart disease, stents
        - CHF
        - Arrhythmia
        - Valve replacement
    - Chronic anticoagulation is a relative contraindication and the decision may be individualized based on circumstances of case
- Obesity with BMI > 40
- Diabetes with A1C > 8–9
- Chronic Anemia with HG < 10
- Substantial OSA
- Renal insufficiency (creatinine > 1.6)
- COPD or pulmonary hypertension
- Chronic liver disease
- Neurologic issues
    - CVA or significant neurologic illness
    - History of frequent falls
    - History of cognitive dysfunction (dementia, Parkinson's)

3. How to successfully perform an outpatient shoulder arthroplasty

3.1 Before surgery

There are several keys to a successful outpatient shoulder arthroplasty. Two of the most important issues surrounding outpatient shoulder arthroplasty are pain control and infection prevention. There are several pieces to pain control including preoperative, intraoperative and postoperative pain management. First, patients undergoing outpatient shoulder arthroplasty are premedicated in the preoperative area prior to surgery. Typically, the authors use 1000 mg of Acetaminophen, 300 mg of Neurontin, and 200 mg of Celecoxib all given orally. The patients are also given regional anesthesia, typically a supraclavicular or interscalene block. The medication used by the anesthesiologist for the block should include a long-acting local anesthetic such as Bupivacaine. Some facilities have moved to using an even longer acting anesthetic such as Bupivacaine liposome injectable suspension (trade name: Exparel), although this can sometimes be cost prohibitive. From an infection prevention perspective, patients are asked to wipe the operative site twice daily with benzoyl peroxide beginning 2 to 3 days prior to surgery and continuing this up until surgery. This helps decrease the C. Acnes load on the skin. Finally, from a timing perspective, it is important to schedule these patients early in the day so they have adequate time to recover before going home. Performing an outpatient arthroplasty later in the day can be tricky and runs the risk that the patient may need to stay overnight.

3.2 Intraoperative

Once the patient has received their block and preoperative medications they are brought back to the operating room where they are given general anesthesia (**Figure 2**). A general anesthetic allows for muscle relaxation which facilitates exposure during a shoulder arthroplasty. To minimize the amount of time the patient is under anesthesia and to mitigate infection risk, it is important to perform the TSA/RTSA efficiently.

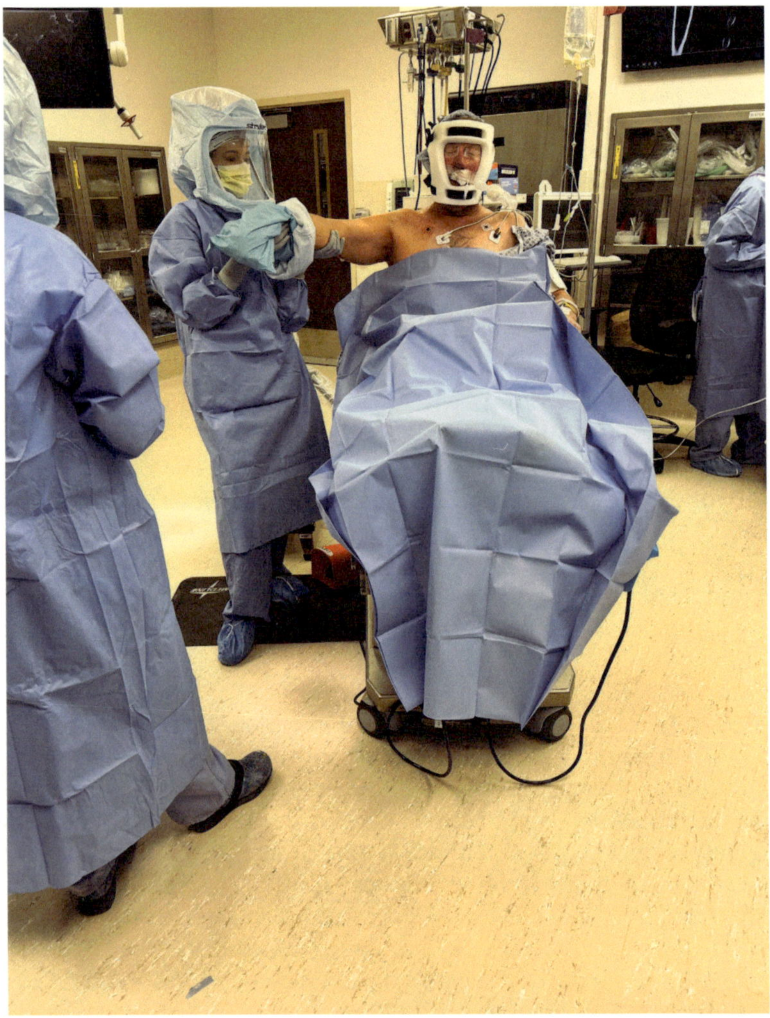

Figure 2.
After general anesthesia, the patient is positioned, draped, and secured in the modified beach chair position.

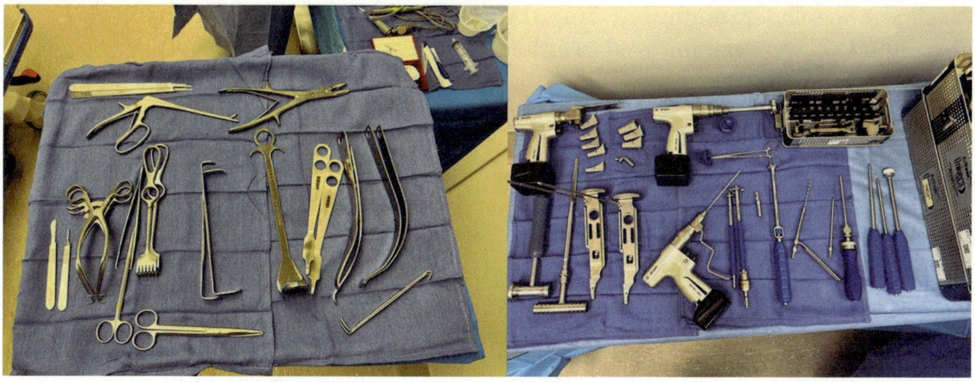

Figure 3.
Instrument and back table organization help expedite the performance of outpatient procedures.

As such, it is important for the surgeon to be comfortable with TSA and RTSA procedures before attempting these in the outpatient setting (**Figure 3**). Having major delays during the procedure keeps the patient under anesthesia for a longer time and may increase the likelihood that they will not go home after surgery. Furthermore, revision TSA/RTSA are not typically performed in the outpatient setting as these patients often have more pain, lose more blood, and have longer operative times than primary cases (**Figure 4**). As surgeons get comfortable with sending patients home the same day following TSA/RTSA, we recommend surgeons perform these cases in an inpatient setting to begin with and send the patients home the same day. Once they have successfully sent these patients home the same day they can progress to performing these cases in the outpatient setting.

Prior to incision the patient should be given 1 g of IV Tranexamic acid (TXA). This acts as a clot stabilizing agent (it is not prothrombotic) and will help minimize blood loss during the procedure. Cvetanovich et al. performed a prospective, double-blind,

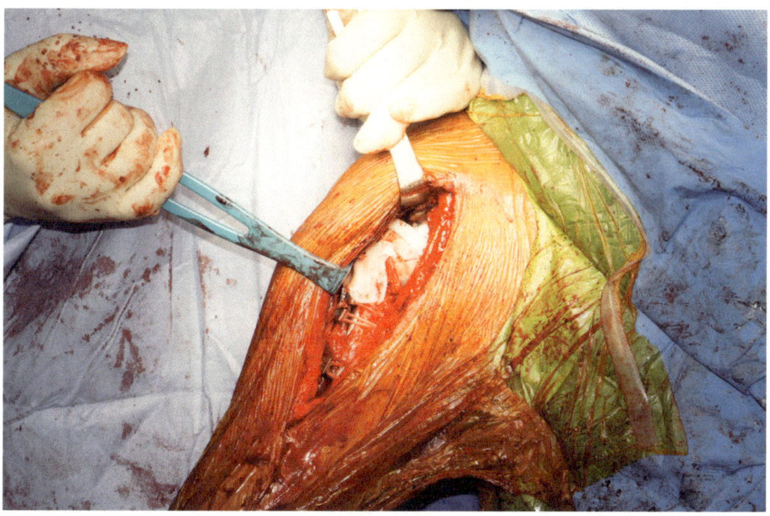

Figure 4.
Revision surgery is usually more complex and demanding. This can require an osteotomy of the humerus that can then be secured with metal or FiberTape cerclages.

placebo-controlled, randomized clinical trial where patients undergoing primary TSA and RTSA were randomized to either receiving 1 g of IV TXA or a placebo to determine if TXA reduced blood loss [8]. The authors included 108 patients (52 for TXA, 56 for placebo) who had no significant differences in preoperative characteristics. They found that the TXA group had significantly lower postoperative blood loss compared with the placebo group. They also found that TXA had lower weight of hemoglobin loss compared with placebo. Similar results were seen in the total knee and total hip arthroplasty literature [9–12]. Similarly, Gillespie et al. randomized 111 patients who underwent shoulder arthroplasty to receive topical saline or topical saline mixed with 2 g of TXA into the wound at the conclusion of the case and measured postoperative drain output (patients at the time of this study all received a drain. This is not done anymore) [13]. The authors found significantly less blood loss in the TXA group compared to the placebo group (108 mL vs. 170 mL) as well as a greater drop in hemoglobin level in the placebo group compared to the TXA group (2.6 g/dL vs. 1.7 g/dL). As such, we routinely use TXA in all of our outpatient shoulder arthroplasty procedures.

Once the preoperative antibiotics (2 g Cefazolin) and Tranexamic acid have been administered, the TSA/RTSA is performed in the standard fashion. The patient is prepped with a hydrogen peroxide wash to decrease the load of C. Acnes on the skin prior to their chlorhexidine prep [14]. The authors use a deltopectoral approach (**Figure 5**). As previously mentioned, exposure is key in TSA and RTSA, so it is important to ensure each layer of dissection is complete to avoid shrinking the operative field. The authors perform a subscapularis peel on all TSA and RTSA (**Figure 6**). Adequate releases on both the humeral and glenoid side will help facilitate glenoid exposure so this is imperative to avoid issues with glenoid pin placement. Once the humeral head cut is made and the glenoid is adequately exposed, the authors use a patient specific guide to place the glenoid pin. A preoperative CT scan is obtained on all patients prior to TSA and RTSA and is unloaded into a preoperative planning software (Virtual Implant Positioning (VIP) Arthrex, Naples FL USA) (**Figure 7**). The ideal glenoid position can then be planned out, and a reusable guide is used to

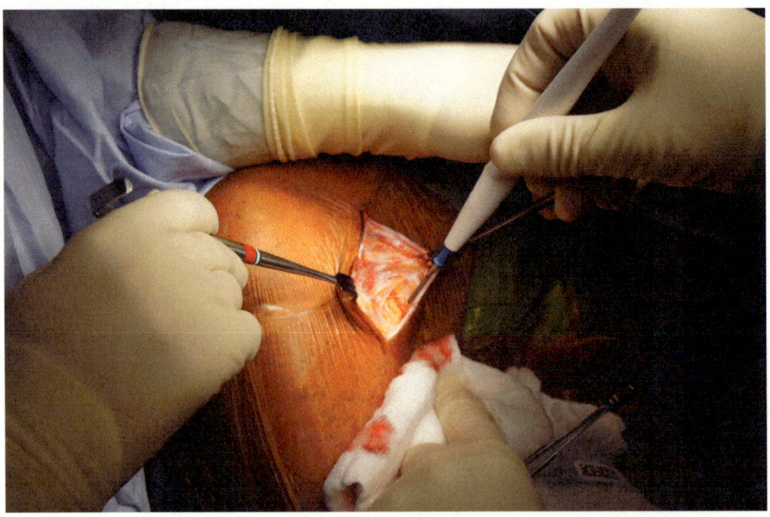

Figure 5.
An example of a deltopectoral incision used in outpatient procedures.

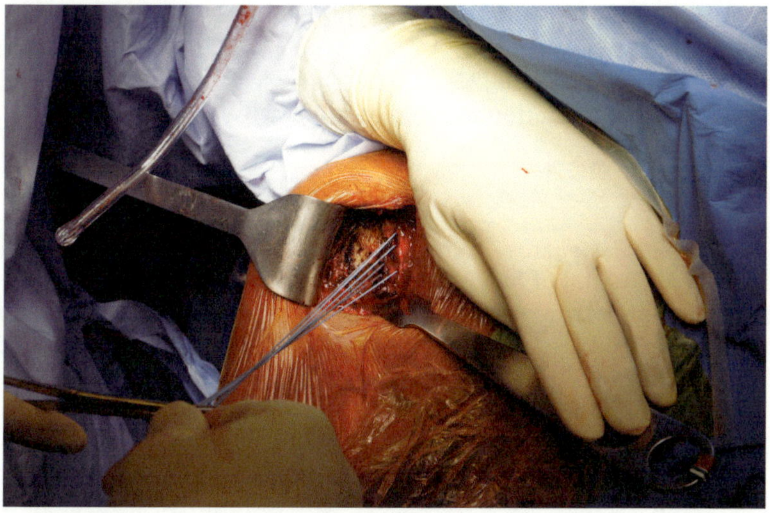

Figure 6.
As part of the optimal visualization, the subscapularis is identified and released from the humerus via a peel technique.

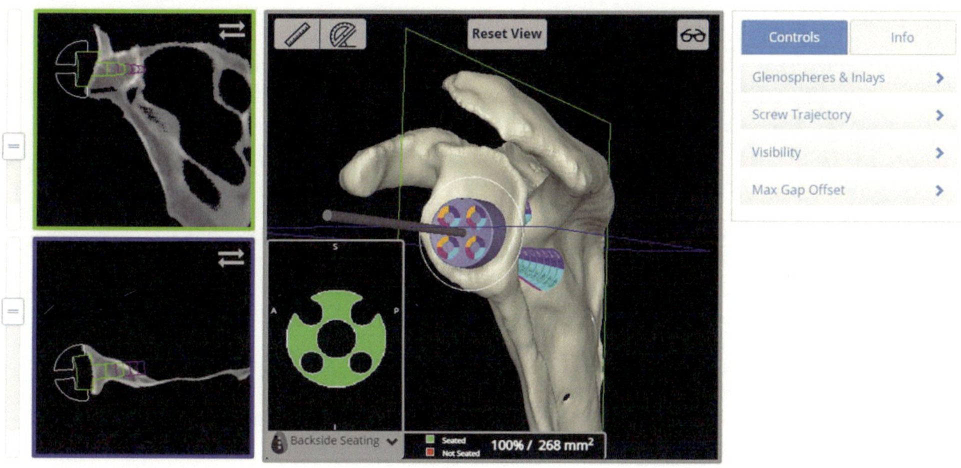

Figure 7.
Preoperative 3D modeling and visualization help execute the surgical plan. This can help minimize the number of trays that need to be available during the procedure.

place the pin in the preoperatively planned position. Once the glenoid component is secured the final humeral implant is placed. The subscapularis is either repaired using a suture anchor repair technique in TSA (SpeedScap, Arthrex, Naples FL, USA) or in transosseous manner with high tensile sutures in RTSA. Based on evidence from the total knee and total hip arthroplasty literature, once the subscapularis has been repaired, it is important to allow the shoulder to soak in dilute betadine for 5 minutes to help decrease the risk of infection [15, 16]. Some surgeons do not allow betadine into operative field as they believe betadine can "burn" tissues. In the author's opinion, this has not been an issue and the addition of betadine has helped mitigate infection risk. Once the dilute betadine has had time to sit it is irrigated out. Next, 1 g of Vancomycin powder is placed in the incision, part just over the subscapularis and part over the deltopectoral closure [17–21]. A running absorbable stitch is used to close the skin along with skin glue. A waterproof silver impregnated dressing is utilized to decrease infection risk [22]. During the case the anesthesia team should ensure adequate patient hydration to avoid postoperative dehydration.

3.3 Postoperative

Following surgery patients are given a set or oral medication including 1000 mg of Acetaminophen, 300 mg of Neurontin, and 200 mg of Celecoxib. If patients are experiencing pain, medications including ketorolac, oxycodone, or tramadol can be utilized on an as needed basis. Ondansetron should be used to control postoperative nausea. A second dose of IV TXA can be given in the recovery room before discharge. A second dose of antibiotics (2 g Cefazolin) is not routinely used unless it has been more than 8 hours since the preoperative dose and the patient has not gone home. Patients are not sent home with any antibiotics. Patients are sent home with a multimodal pain regimen. Further work is needed to determine the ideal combination of medications, but some of the options to include are: Acetaminophen, Tramadol, Oxycodone, Gabapentin, Celecoxib, Aspirin and Pantoprazole.

3.4 Physical therapy

The demand for shoulder arthroplasty is projected to exceed that of hip/knee arthroplasty [23]. For instance, it has been reported that a total of 39,072 patients were admitted for total shoulder arthroplasty in 2010, 5 times the number of patients in 1998 [24]. This increase is proportionally associated with the need for effective and feasible physical therapy, which is critical in the recovery pathway following shoulder replacements [25]. Traditionally, physical therapy following shoulder surgery has occurred via in-office supervised visits [26]. Home-based physical therapy reduces costs and decreases the need for travel [27]. Home-based therapy has been shown to be as effective as in-office therapy after total knee arthroplasty and has been utilized for rehabilitation after proximal humerus fracture [28–30]. It has also been reported to be a safe and effective alternative in the early phase following rotator cuff repair [31]. However, home-based therapy lacks the ability to monitor patient performance, compliance, and progress. Digital health has been incorporated in various medical fields over the past few decades. This process has accelerated since the COVID-19 pandemic which has brought to the forefront of medicine the need to deliver care and rehabilitation remotely. Remote patient monitoring has emerged as a concept in which patient physiologic parameters are measured and remotely delivered to a care team. Within our practice, remote patient monitoring is implemented via a secure cloud-based provider rehabilitation platform that communicates with a patient application powered by marker-less artificial intelligence (AI) technology with a dedicated built-in telemedicine capability (PT Genie; Orlando, FL) (**Figure 8**).

At the initial visit patients are instructed on how to use the platform and are provided a QR code to scan and download the app onto their device (Android/iOS). PT Genie has instructions on the home-based exercise protocol, demonstrates the exercises to be performed and keeps track of progress including pain score, completed repetitions and number of sessions all via the AI driven sensor less motion tracking using the front facing camera of a cellphone or a tablet. Monitoring is performed on

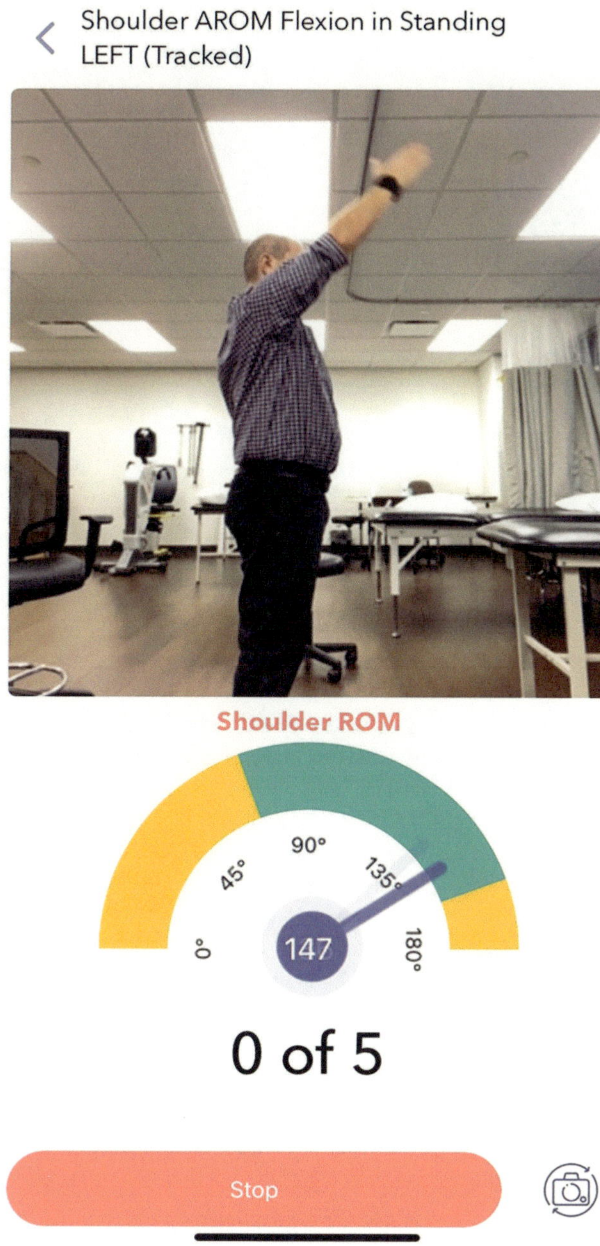

Figure 8.
The patient-facing application (PT Genie) which tacks ROM using AI marker less technology.

the web-based clinical dashboard by a dedicated care team, who also monitor the daily progress and communicate with the patients via in-app messages, telemedicine calls, and emails (**Figure 9**). PT Genie allows the provider to fully customize and control the rehabilitation protocol by adding or modifying exercises to go along with the patient's pace of recovery, the addition of bands and calculation of force on certain exercises, and the ability to set up a pre habilitation phase, if needed prior to surgery.

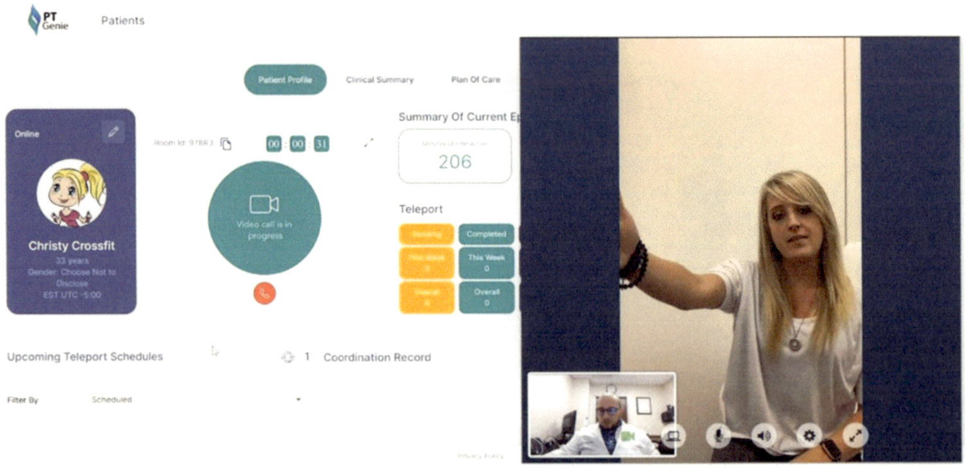

Figure 9.
A secure telemedicine platform (PT Genie) enables the provider and the patient to communicate and interact remotely.

4. Results of outpatient shoulder arthroplasty

Several studies have shown the efficacy of outpatient TSA and RTSA compared to inpatient shoulder arthroplasty. Cimino et al. performed a systematic review of 12 studies (194,513 patients, of whom 7162 were outpatients) to evaluate the outcomes following outpatient TSA and RTSA [32]. The average age of the outpatients was 66.6 years while the average age of the inpatients was 70.1 years. The authors found the odds ratio for complications was significantly lower in outpatients than in inpatients. Furthermore, there was no significant difference in rates of 90-day readmission, revision, and infection rate between outpatients with inpatients. Similarly, Fournier et al. reported the results of 61 patients who underwent outpatient TSA and RTSA [6]. There were no cardiopulmonary events that required intervention or hospital admission. These studies evaluated both TSA and RTSA together. This happens commonly because the CPT code for TSA and RTSA is the same (23472). Below are examples of studies that separated outcome based on TSA and RTSA.

i. TSA

Erickson et al. reported the results of 94 patients (average age 60.4, 67.0% male) who underwent TSA 2015–2017 by the senior author. The authors matched this group of patients to a group of 77 patients who underwent TSA as an inpatient. Patients who underwent outpatient TSA saw significant improvement in all clinical outcome scores at both 1 and 2 year postoperatively (**Figure 10**). There were baseline differences between groups such that patients who underwent inpatient TSA were more likely to be diabetic than those who underwent outpatient TSA. The authors found no significant differences in improvements in clinical outcome scores between inpatients vs. outpatient groups. They noted that complications were more frequent in patients who underwent inpatient TSA (11.4% vs. 2.1%), although this did difference did not reach statistical significance ($p = 0.080$). Brolin et al. evaluated 30 patients who underwent outpatient TSA at a freestanding ambulatory surgery center and compared

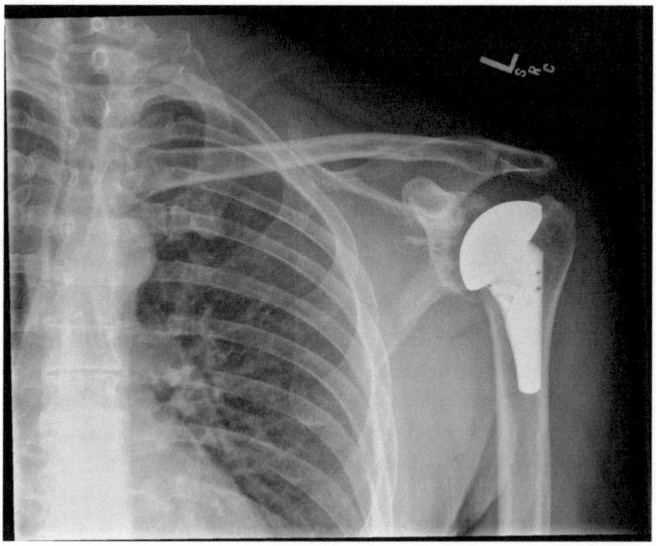

Figure 10.
A 2-years follow-up X-ray for an outpatient total shoulder arthroplasty (TSA).

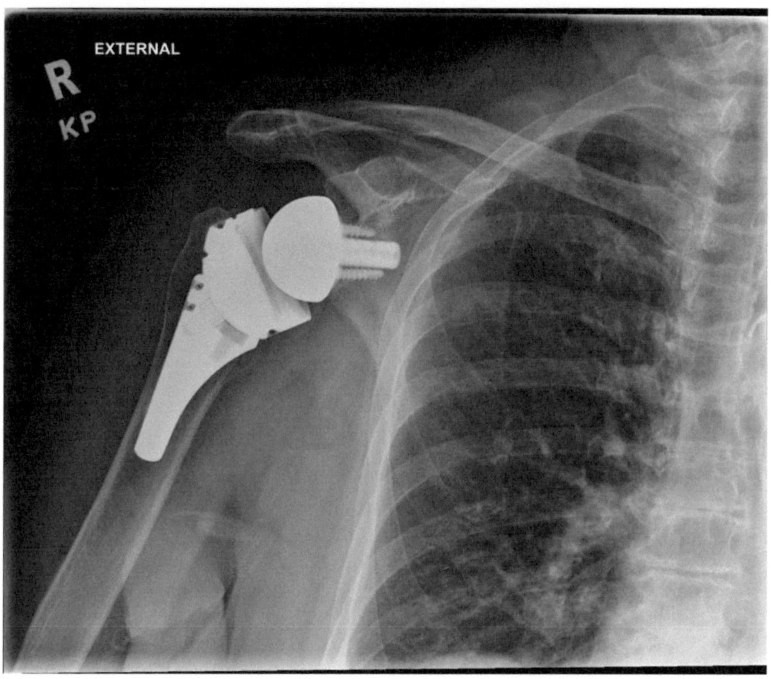

Figure 11.
A 2-years follow-up X-ray for an outpatient reverse total shoulder arthroplasty (RTSA).

them with an age- and comorbidities-matched cohort of 30 patients who underwent inpatient TSA [5]. The authors evaluated 90-day complications, hospital admissions/readmissions and reoperations. There were significant differences between outpatient and inpatient cohorts regarding preoperative demographics. The authors reported no hospital admissions from the outpatient cohort and no readmissions from the inpatient cohort. There was no difference in the complication rates between outpatient (13%) and inpatient (10%) shoulder arthroplasty.

ii. RTSA.

Erickson et al. reported the results on 241 patients (average age 68.9, 52.3% female) who underwent outpatient RTSA between 2015 and 2017 by the senior author (**Figure 11**). The authors matched this group of patients to a group of 373 patients who underwent RTSA as an inpatient. There were baseline differences between the two groups such that significantly more inpatient RTSA had diabetes ($p = 0.007$) and had a significantly higher body mass index ($p = 0.022$). The authors found that patients who underwent outpatient RTSA had significant improvement in all clinical outcome scores at both 1 and 2 year postoperatively (all $p < 0.0001$). There were no significant differences in improvements in clinical outcome scores between inpatient vs. outpatient RTSA groups. Most importantly, complication rates were significantly lower for patients who underwent RSTA as an outpatient compared to those who underwent RTSA as an inpatient (7.0% vs. 12.7% $p = 0.023$).

5. Conclusion

Many patients are candidates for outpatient TSA and RTSA. Some patients may be better suited to have their surgery performed in the hospital setting while other are excellent candidates for an outpatient surgical center. A thorough preoperative evaluation is critical for proper patient selection and a set protocol is necessary for the day of surgery to ensure proper pain control and to minimize risk of complications and readmissions. When performed properly, patients should expect the same outcomes as those who undergo TSA and RTSA in the inpatient setting with potentially lower complication rates.

Author details

Brandon J. Erickson[1]*, Yousef Shishani[2] and Reuben Gobezie[2]

1 Rothman Orthopaedic Institute, New York, USA

2 Cleveland Shoulder Institute, Beachwood, OH, USA

*Address all correspondence to: brandon.erickson@rothmanortho.com

References

[1] Erickson BJ, Bohl DD, Cole BJ, et al. Reverse total shoulder arthroplasty: Indications and techniques across the world. American Journal of Orthopedics (Belle Mead, N.J.). 2018;**47**(9). DOI: 10.12788/ajo.2018.0079

[2] Gupta AK, Harris JD, Erickson BJ, et al. Surgical management of complex proximal humerus fractures -A systematic review of 92 studies including 4,500 patients. Journal of Orthopaedic Trauma. 2015;**29**(1):54-59

[3] Hadley CSN, Anis H, Ricchetti E, Mont MA, Erickson BJ, Romeo AA. Nationwide trends of surgical site infections rates after primary shoulder arthroplasty. Seminars in Arthroplasty: JSES. 2021;**31**(2):191-196

[4] Basques BA, Erickson BJ, Leroux T, et al. Comparative outcomes of outpatient and inpatient total shoulder arthroplasty: An analysis of the Medicare dataset. The Bone & Joint Journal. 2017;**99-B**(7):934-938

[5] Brolin TJ, Mulligan RP, Azar FM, Throckmorton TW. Neer Award 2016: Outpatient total shoulder arthroplasty in an ambulatory surgery center is a safe alternative to inpatient total shoulder arthroplasty in a hospital: A matched cohort study. Journal of Shoulder and Elbow Surgery. 2017;**26**(2):204-208

[6] Fournier MN, Brolin TJ, Azar FM, Stephens R, Throckmorton TW. Identifying appropriate candidates for ambulatory outpatient shoulder arthroplasty: Validation of a patient selection algorithm. Journal of Shoulder and Elbow Surgery. 2019;**28**(1):65-70

[7] Leroux TS, Basques BA, Frank RM, et al. Outpatient total shoulder arthroplasty: A population-based study comparing adverse event and readmission rates to inpatient total shoulder arthroplasty. Journal of Shoulder and Elbow Surgery. 2016;**25**(11):1780-1786

[8] Cvetanovich GL, Fillingham YA, O'Brien M, et al. Tranexamic acid reduces blood loss after primary shoulder arthroplasty: A double-blind, placebo-controlled, prospective, randomized controlled trial. JSES Open Access. 2018;**2**(1):23-27

[9] Fillingham YA, Darrith B, Calkins TE, et al. Mark Coventry Award: A multicentre randomized clinical trial of tranexamic acid in revision total knee arthroplasty: Does the dosing regimen matter? The Bone & Joint Journal. 2019;**101-B**(7_Supple_C):10-16

[10] Fillingham YA, Ramkumar DB, Jevsevar DS, et al. Tranexamic acid in total joint arthroplasty: The endorsed clinical practice guides of the American Association of Hip and Knee Surgeons, American Society of Regional Anesthesia and Pain Medicine, American Academy of Orthopaedic Surgeons, Hip Society, and Knee Society. Regional Anesthesia and Pain Medicine. 2019;**44**(1):7-11

[11] Fillingham YA, Ramkumar DB, Jevsevar DS, et al. The efficacy of tranexamic acid in total knee arthroplasty: A network meta-analysis. The Journal of Arthroplasty. 2018;**33**(10):3090-3098 e3091

[12] Kayupov E, Fillingham YA, Okroj K, et al. Oral and intravenous tranexamic acid are equivalent at reducing blood loss following total hip arthroplasty: A randomized controlled trial. The Journal of Bone and Joint Surgery. American Volume. 2017;**99**(5):373-378

[13] Gillespie R, Shishani Y, Joseph S, Streit JJ, Gobezie R. Neer Award 2015: A randomized, prospective evaluation on the effectiveness of tranexamic acid in reducing blood loss after total shoulder arthroplasty. Journal of Shoulder and Elbow Surgery. 2015;**24**(11):1679-1684

[14] Chalmers PN, Beck L, Stertz I, Tashjian RZ. Hydrogen peroxide skin preparation reduces Cutibacterium acnes in shoulder arthroplasty: A prospective, blinded, controlled trial. Journal of Shoulder and Elbow Surgery. 2019;**28**(8):1554-1561

[15] Brown NM, Cipriano CA, Moric M, Sporer SM, Della Valle CJ. Dilute betadine lavage before closure for the prevention of acute postoperative deep periprosthetic joint infection. The Journal of Arthroplasty. 2012;**27**(1):27-30

[16] Calkins TE, Culvern C, Nam D, et al. Dilute betadine lavage reduces the risk of acute postoperative periprosthetic joint infection in aseptic revision total knee and hip arthroplasty: A randomized controlled trial. The Journal of Arthroplasty. 2020;**35**(2):538-543 e531

[17] Buchalter DB, Kirby DJ, Teo GM, Iorio R, Aggarwal VK, Long WJ. Topical vancomycin powder and dilute povidone-iodine lavage reduce the rate of early periprosthetic joint infection after primary total knee arthroplasty. The Journal of Arthroplasty. 2021;**36**(1): 286-290 e281

[18] Hatch MD, Daniels SD, Glerum KM, Higgins LD. The cost effectiveness of vancomycin for preventing infections after shoulder arthroplasty: A break-even analysis. Journal of Shoulder and Elbow Surgery. 2017;**26**(3):472-477

[19] Hosack LW, Overstreet DJ, Lederman ES. In vitro susceptibility of *Propionibacterium acnes* to simulated intrawound vancomycin concentrations. JSES Open Access. 2017;**1**(3):125-128

[20] Iorio R, Yu S, Anoushiravani AA, et al. Vancomycin powder and dilute povidone-iodine lavage for infection prophylaxis in high-risk total joint arthroplasty. The Journal of Arthroplasty. 2020;**35**(7):1933-1936

[21] Miquel J, Huang TB, Athwal GS, Faber KJ, O'Gorman DB. Vancomycin is effective in preventing *Cutibacterium acnes* growth in a mimetic shoulder arthroplasty. Journal of Shoulder and Elbow Surgery. 2021;**31**(1):159-164

[22] Grosso MJ, Berg A, LaRussa S, Murtaugh T, Trofa DP, Geller JA. Silver-impregnated occlusive dressing reduces rates of acute periprosthetic joint infection after total joint arthroplasty. The Journal of Arthroplasty. 2017;**32**(3): 929-932

[23] Day JS, Lau E, Ong KL, Williams GR, Ramsey ML, Kurtz SM. Prevalence and projections of total shoulder and elbow arthroplasty in the United States to 2015. Journal of Shoulder and Elbow Surgery. 2010;**19**(8):1115-1120

[24] Issa K, Pierce CM, Pierce TP, et al. Total shoulder arthroplasty demographics, incidence, and complications-A nationwide inpatient sample database study. Surgical Technology International. 2016;**29**:240-246

[25] Christiansen DH, Frost P, Falla D, et al. Effectiveness of standardized physical therapy exercises for patients with difficulty returning to usual activities after decompression surgery for subacromial impingement syndrome: Randomized controlled trial. Physical Therapy. 2016;**96**(6):787-796

[26] Arshi A, Kabir N, Cohen JR, et al. Utilization and costs of postoperative

physical therapy after rotator cuff repair: A comparison of privately insured and medicare patients. Arthroscopy. 2015;**31**(12):2392-2399 e2391

[27] Pastora-Bernal JM, Martin-Valero R, Baron-Lopez FJ, Estebanez-Perez MJ. Evidence of benefit of telerehabitation after orthopedic surgery: A systematic review. Journal of Medical Internet Research. 2017;**19**(4):e142

[28] Moffet H, Tousignant M, Nadeau S, et al. In-home telerehabilitation compared with face-to-face rehabilitation after total knee arthroplasty: A noninferiority randomized controlled trial. The Journal of Bone and Joint Surgery. American Volume. 2015;**97**(14):1129-1141

[29] Piqueras M, Marco E, Coll M, et al. Effectiveness of an interactive virtual telerehabilitation system in patients after total knee arthoplasty: A randomized controlled trial. Journal of Rehabilitation Medicine. 2013;**45**(4):392-396

[30] Tousignant M, Giguere AM, Morin M, Pelletier J, Sheehy A, Cabana F. In-home telerehabilitation for proximal humerus fractures: A pilot study. International Journal of Telerehabilitation. 2014;**6**(2):31-37

[31] Buvik A, Bergmo TS, Bugge E, Smaabrekke A, Wilsgaard T, Olsen JA. Cost-effectiveness of telemedicine in remote orthopedic consultations: Randomized controlled trial. Journal of Medical Internet Research. 2019;**21**(2): e11330

[32] Cimino AM, Hawkins JK, McGwin G, Brabston EW, Ponce BA, Momaya AM. Is outpatient shoulder arthroplasty safe? A systematic review and meta-analysis. Journal of Shoulder and Elbow Surgery. 2021;**30**(8):1968-1976

Section 3

Shoulder Tumors and Dyskinesis

Chapter 6

Shoulder Surgery for Bone Tumors

Stephanie D. Zarate and Ana C. Belzarena

Abstract

The proximal humerus is a common location for bone tumors. Those can affect patients of different ages and can be of benign or malignant nature. For bone sarcomas is the 3rd most common location and is a frequent site of spread in non-axial metastatic disease. In pediatric patients is frequent to encounter benign bone tumors in this location but also osteosarcomas and Ewing's sarcomas. Careful assessment of the patients by a surgeon with the appropriate training is paramount. Shoulder reconstruction for patients with bone tumors encompasses a diverse group of patients, diagnoses and surgical options. While most patients with primary bone tumors may be of a younger age and more involved in sport activities, those with metastatic disease oftentimes are associated with an older age, worse preoperative function and worse prognosis due to the primary disease. The surgeon must weigh in all factors that need to be taken into consideration in the treatment decision-making plan. Currently, with new advances in oncology treatments patients may benefit from longer survivals times than in the past, thus restoring the patient's function and quality of life is essential.

Keywords: shoulder surgery, bone tumors, sarcoma, metastatic disease, shoulder reconstruction

1. Introduction

The proximal humerus is a common location for bone tumors, benign and malignant, in all age ranges [1–3]. For bone sarcomas is the 3rd most common location and is a frequent site of spread in non-axial metastatic disease [2]. The most common primary tumors to cause bone secondary lesions are breast, prostate and lung usually through a mechanism of hematogenous spread [4]. In the pediatric population benign tumors outnumber the malignant ones, with osteochondromas and enchondromas being the most frequent [5]. Primary malignant bone tumors are more common at a younger age, with osteosarcoma being the most common followed by Ewing's sarcoma [6]. While most benign primary bone tumors tend to be asymptomatic and usually diagnosed as an incidental finding, malignant tumors are more likely to cause symptoms. Pain constitutes the main complaint followed by tenderness locally and swelling of the soft tissues. The pain located over the affected bone can be nocturnal, present at rest or constant, of progressive intensity and more or less resistant to over-the-counter pain medication [7]. Malignant and aggressive tumors that remain long periods undiagnosed or without treatment may progress to a pathological fracture, event occurring in up to 10% of osteosarcomas [8]. In the case of metastatic disease, it is an ominous sign and carries a poor prognosis and increased mortality [9].

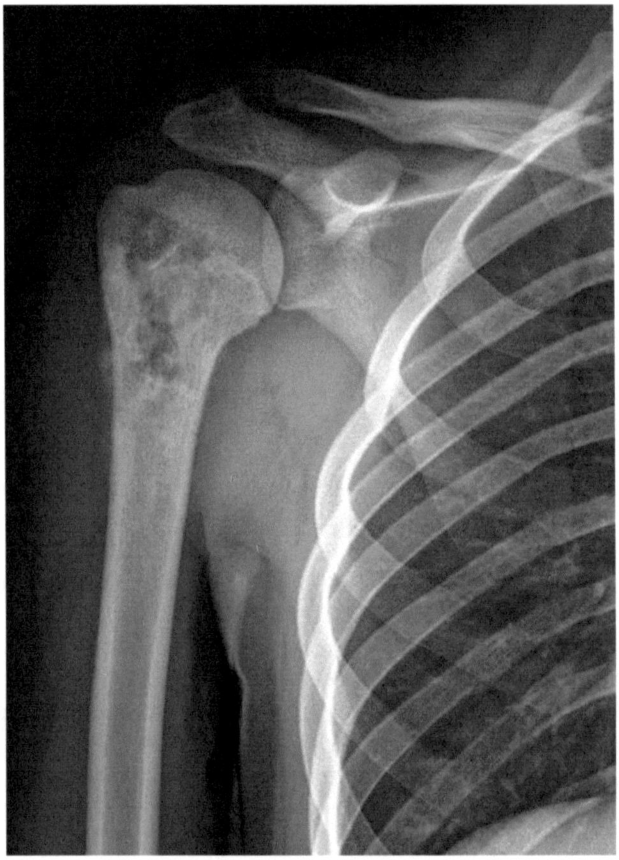

Figure 1.
Antero-posterior radiograph of a 17-year-old patient with a destructive lesion of the proximal right humerus with a mixed patter, of lytic lesions and osteoid production, and periosteal reaction.

When patients present initially without a diagnosis the first step is obtaining a thorough history and performing a detailed physical examination, with emphasis on the shoulder function. Following imaging studies need to be obtained. The first imaging exam is a radiograph of the shoulder as well as the humerus (**Figure 1**). The orthopedic surgeon should assess for the type of lesion; if it is blastic, lytic or mixed; its limits, the presence of periosteal reaction, associated soft tissue masses or a pathological fracture (**Figure 2**). Computed tomography can also be obtained to assess the cortical integrity of the bone and for surgical planning as well (**Figure 3**). Additionally computed tomography can show calcifications, healing response in case of pathological fractures and are useful for biopsy guidance as well. The biopsy tract when performed by a physician other than the surgeon should be discussed with the surgeon performing the definitive treatment [10].

In cases where a primary bone sarcoma is suspected a magnetic resonance should be obtained with and without contrast (**Figure 4**). The entirety of the bone must be imaged due to the occasional presence of skip lesions [11]. In the case where metastatic disease is suspected or for staging purposes of a primary sarcoma, a bone scan should be obtained to assess for additional bone lesions (**Figure 5**).

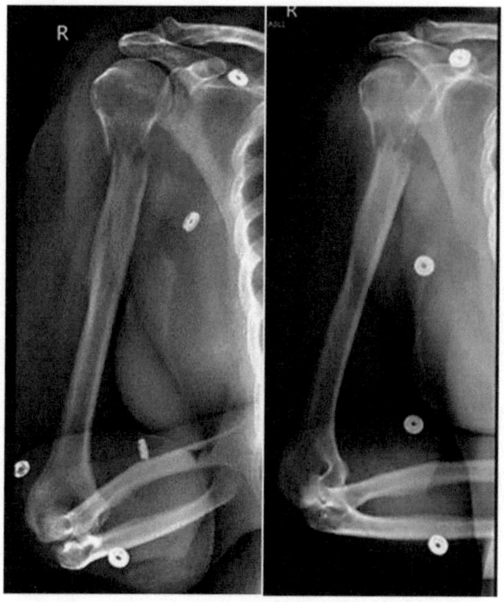

Figure 2.
Radiographic images, anterior–posterior and lateral of proximal right humerus lytic lesion and pathological fracture in a lung cancer patient.

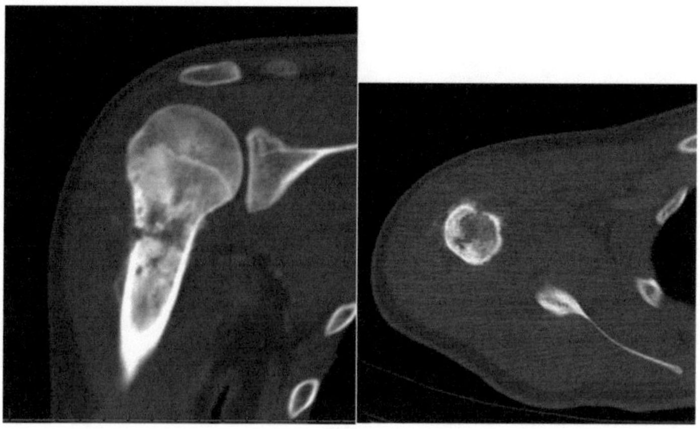

Figure 3.
Coronal and axial view of a proximal humerus computed tomography without contrast depicting an aggressive-appearing destructive lesion that has eroded through the cortex.

Once a diagnosis has been made the treatment plan needs to be formulated. The goal of surgery will depend on the diagnosis, benign versus malignant, primary versus secondary lesion. In the case of benign lesions surgical treatment is usually reserved for symptomatic patients, for example in the case of an osteochondroma impinging at the extremes of range of motion. For metastatic lesions the goal is to render a pain free and functional patient, taking into consideration the overall prognosis of the disease. For primary bone sarcomas, the mainstay of treatment is surgical resection with adequate margins and a functional reconstruction, preferably performed by a surgeon with experience on sarcoma care [12].

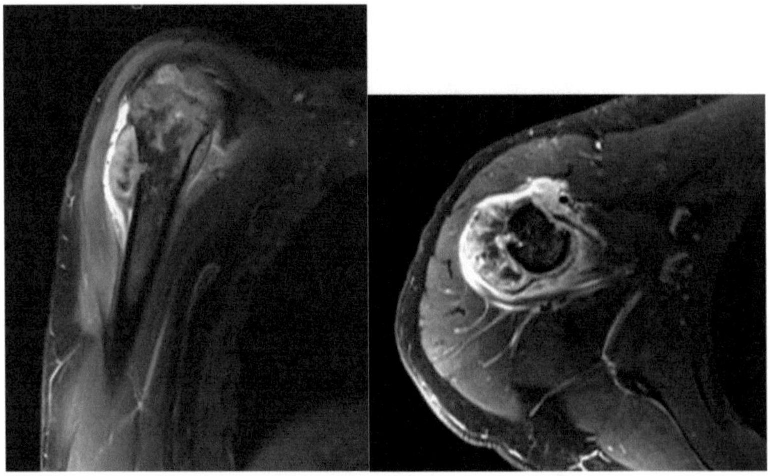

Figure 4.
Magnetic resonance of the humerus with and without gadolinium enhancement. Coronal and axial T1-fat-suppresed with contrast sequence depicting a proximal humerus bone sarcoma with associated surrounding soft tissue component.

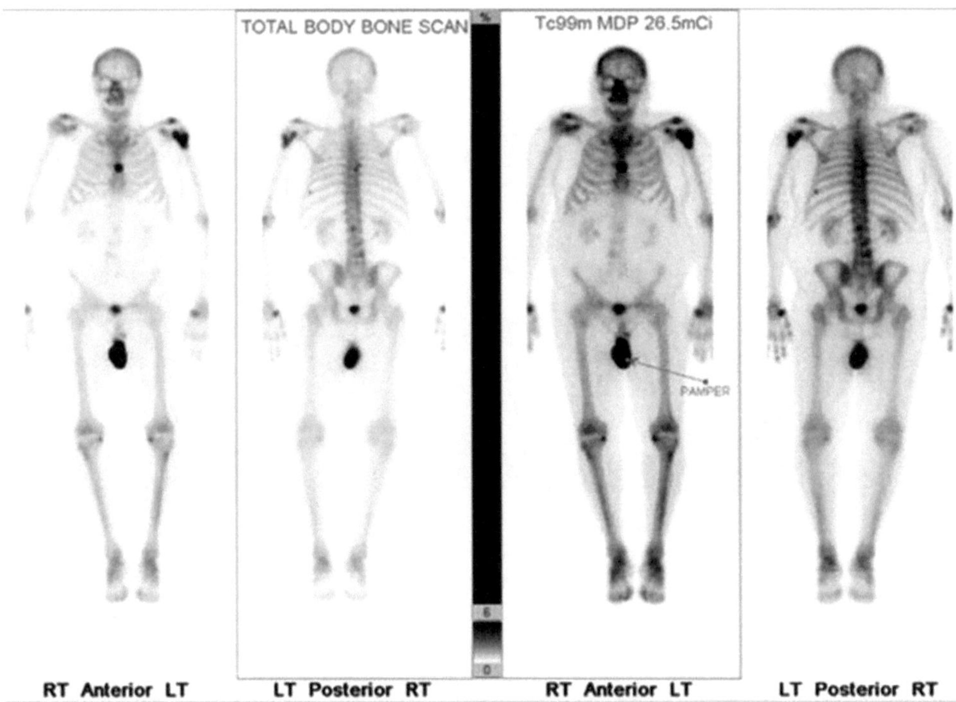

Figure 5.
Bone scintigraphy study with Tecnecium-99 depicting a lesion in the proximal left humerus and sternum.

2. Internal fixation for metastatic disease of the proximal Humerus

After assessing the lesion characteristics and the patient's overall prognosis, a decision has to be made regarding the surgical planning. For widely metastatic disease and

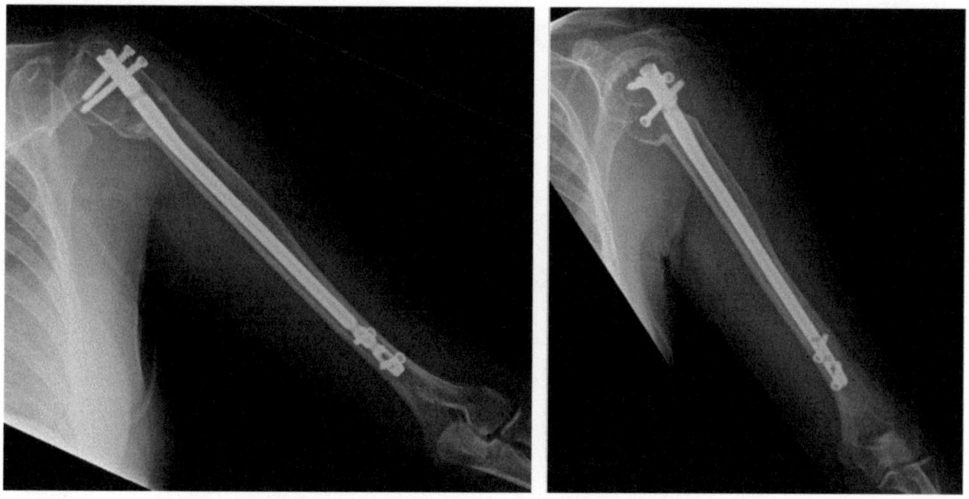

Figure 6.
Radiograph depicting disease progression of a metastatic lesion in the proximal humerus and bony destruction.

a pathological fracture of the proximal metadiaphyseal region internal fixation can be indicated. Intramedullary nailing or a proximal plate and screws are valid options. Both procedures are performed according to the traditional technique and approach. Depending on the location and extent of the lesion, curettage and cement augmentation may be incorporated into the procedure as a means of enhancing disease local control and implant survival. A novel device composed of a liquid photodynamic monomer is an additional alternative providing strength and stability under rotational forces [13]. The advantage of long intramedullary devices in patients with metastatic disease is the protection of the entire bone in the event of further disease progression. Radiotherapy is often indicated postoperatively to increase local disease control [14]. In the event of disease progression, the fixation implant may fail requiring a second, potentially more morbid, surgical procedure for revision (**Figure 6**).

3. Proximal Humerus resection and reconstruction

Primary bone malignancy as well as extensive secondary disease with poor bone stock may require a bone resection followed by reconstruction. In the decision-making process is important to take into account the diagnosis, the patient's prognosis as well as the structures involved by the tumor which may need to be resected along the bone such as the rotator cuff or the axillary nerve. For proximal humerus tumors the approach is usually the delto-pectoral approach including the biopsy tract, slightly lateral to the delto-pectoral line, with the resection specimen in the case of primary tumors. The surrounding structures involved and included in the resection will determine the postoperative function of the patient and will dictate the type of reconstruction indicated. When both the rotator cuff and an innervated deltoid muscle can be preserved allograph-prostheses composite can be used. If only a functional deltoid is maintained but the rotator cuff is involved in the resection, a reverse total shoulder can be used for the reconstruction. For tumors extending outside of the humerus where the deltoid and rotator cuff have to be resected, a proximal humerus endoprosthesis can be used as a spacer (**Figure 7**).

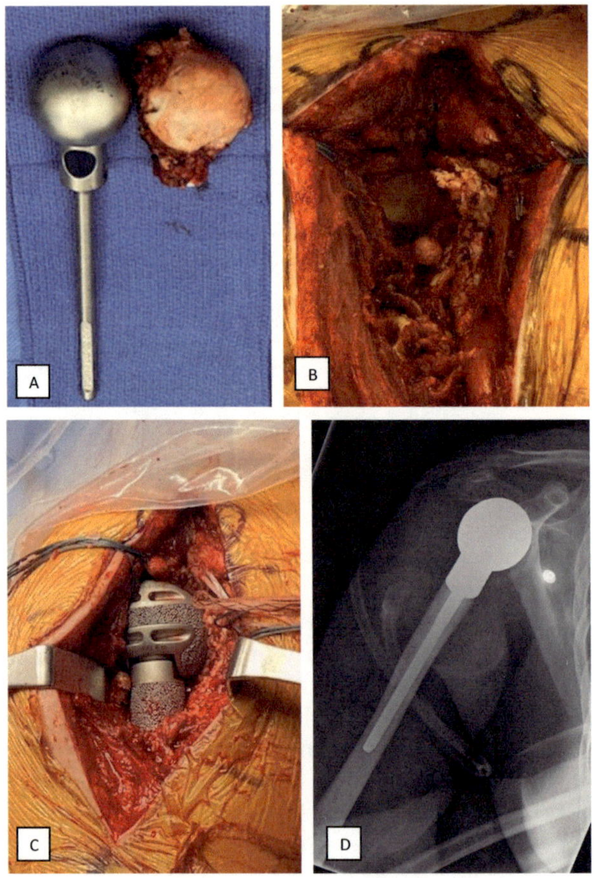

Figure 7.
Clinical images and radiographs of a proximal humerus resection. A: Resection piece and trial implant. B: Surrounding soft tissues remaining tagged. C: Implant in place, tagged from the surrounding soft tissues are later attached to the implant. D: Final radiograph showing the implant in place, a long stem was chosen given the presence of metastatic lesions distally.

For proximal humerus tumor resection and reconstruction the complication rate ranges from 20 to 45% [15]. Dislocation of the implant along infection are the most common encountered problems (**Figure 8**). Besides any hardware or surgically related complications, local recurrences can be another problematic event for these patients. Occurring in 12% of patients, tumor recurrences are a common cause for a subsequent amputation [16]. For surgical constructs where an allograft is added or used as a reconstruction option, the most common complications are fracture, infection and collapse of the subchondral surface [17, 18]. Comparing the diverse options for tumor resection, endoprosthetic replacement is the one associated with lowest complication rates whereas allograft-implant composites would have a better functional outcome [19]. Some authors advocate for the use of a vascular synthetic mesh around the implant for proximal humerus endoprosthetic reconstructions to reduce the rate of dislocations [20, 21]. The mesh creates a surface for adherence of the remaining surrounding soft tissue attachments (**Figure 9**). For a small percentage of patients, resection and reconstruction may not be an option and an amputation will have to be indicated, fortunately due to advances in surgical implants as well as adjuvant treatments such as radiotherapy and chemotherapy, most patients can benefit from a limb

DOI: http://dx.doi.org/10.5772/intechopen.102746

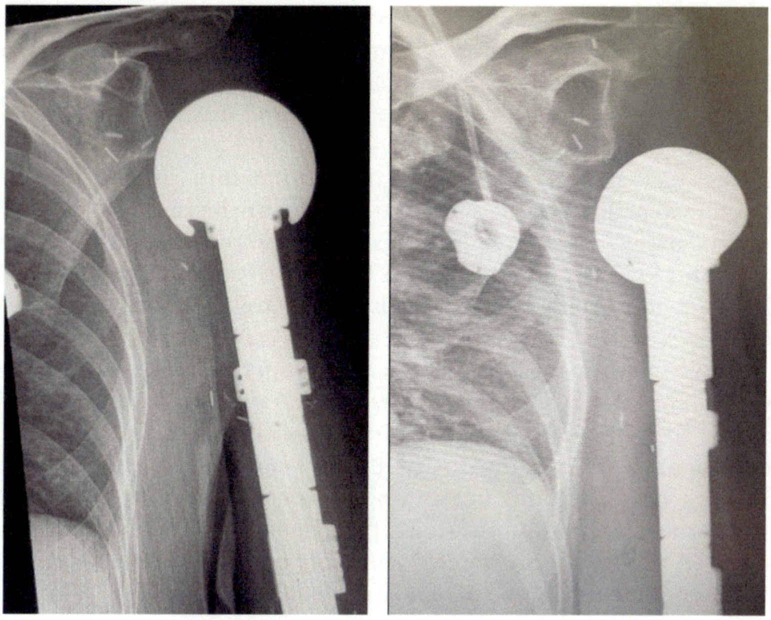

Figure 8.
Radiographic image depicting a dislocated humeral endoprostheses, one of the most common complications.

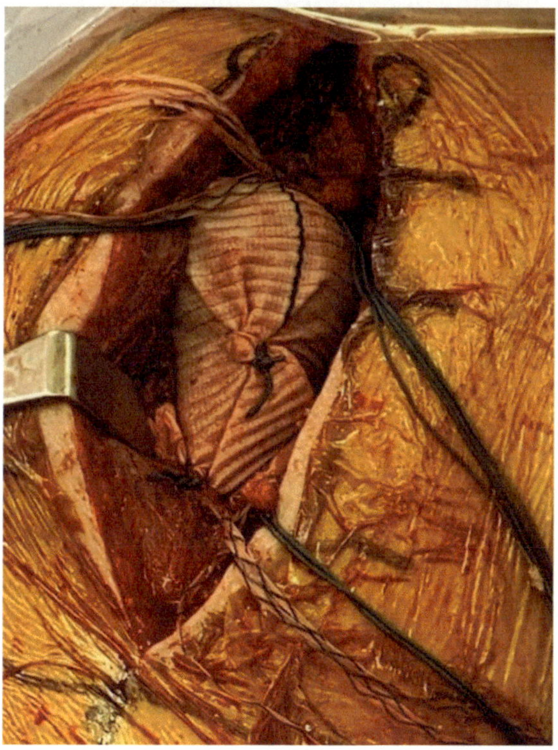

Figure 9.
Clinical image of a proximal humerus endoprosthetic replacement with surrounding vascular synthetic mesh and surrounding soft tissues tagged for later reattachment to the mesh.

salvage procedure [22]. In cases where the tumor extends into the glenohumeral joint or even into the scapula a Tikhoff-Linberg amputation may be indicated. This procedure consists of an extra-articular resection of all the areas involved by the tumor plus a surrounding adequate surgical margin [23]. This procedure has been associated with high rate of complications and mortality [24, 25].

Prior studies have shown that the implant survivorship for proximal humerus replacement due to primary bone sarcomas is 77% for the first year and 74% at 5 years from the index procedure [26]. Most common reasons for implant failure are infections and local tumor recurrences [26]. The functional outcomes for these patients are going to be determined by the reconstruction type but also by the extent of the resection and the structures involved. The activity level has been shown to decrease significantly in the first year from the initial operation with some improvement after 3 years, yet to lower levels than preoperatively [27]. Moreover, even though most patients remain active and are able to get back and be involved in sport activities, most patients have to switch to a lower extremity activity such as soccer, bicycling or running. Those who prior to surgery practiced sports with overhead activities, unfortunately are usually not able to return to that sport [27]. A slightly improved level of sport performance can be expected in patients where the resection can spare an active deltoid muscle [28]. Some authors also advocate for the use of the synthetic vascular mesh as a means of increasing shoulder function as well [21].

4. Curettage and grafting of benign and aggressive lesions

The proximal humerus is a common location for benign bone tumors such as osteochondromas, enchondromas and unicameral bone cysts. Additionally, it is also a frequent location for more aggressive lesions such as or chondroblastomas. As with other bone tumors the assessment starts with a thorough history taking and physical examination followed by the appropriate imaging studies. In questionable cases or where imaging findings are non-specific a biopsy is indicated, performed ideally by a physician with the appropriate training on bone tumors. For most benign lesions patients are asymptomatic and diagnosis is made incidentally. Non-aggressive lesions such as non-ossifying fibromas, asymptomatic osteochondromas or enchondromas, observation may be all the necessary treatment. Curettage is indicated in the case of aggressive bone tumors that tend to continue to grow causing bone destruction or even a pathological fracture. Others such as atypical cartilaginous tumors may later on dedifferentiate into a higher-grade tumor [29]. The surgery usually involved a small incision over the most direct pathway to the lesion. Once the bone is reached a small window is created with the help of a burr or an osteotome. The lesion is thoroughly and carefully curetted avoiding any spilling of the surrounding tissues. Fluoroscopic visualization may help confirm all the extent of the lesion has been reached (**Figure 10**). In the case of unicameral bone cysts, intramedullary decompression with the help of a curette or a Kirschner wire of the canal is indicated [30]. In the case of aggressive lesions, the use of adjuvants such as nitrogen, phenol or high-speed burr can help decrease the local recurrence, a common outcome for these type of tumors [31]. Once the lesion has been curetted there are several options for filling such as autologous bone graft, allografts and synthetic bone substitutes (**Figure 10**).

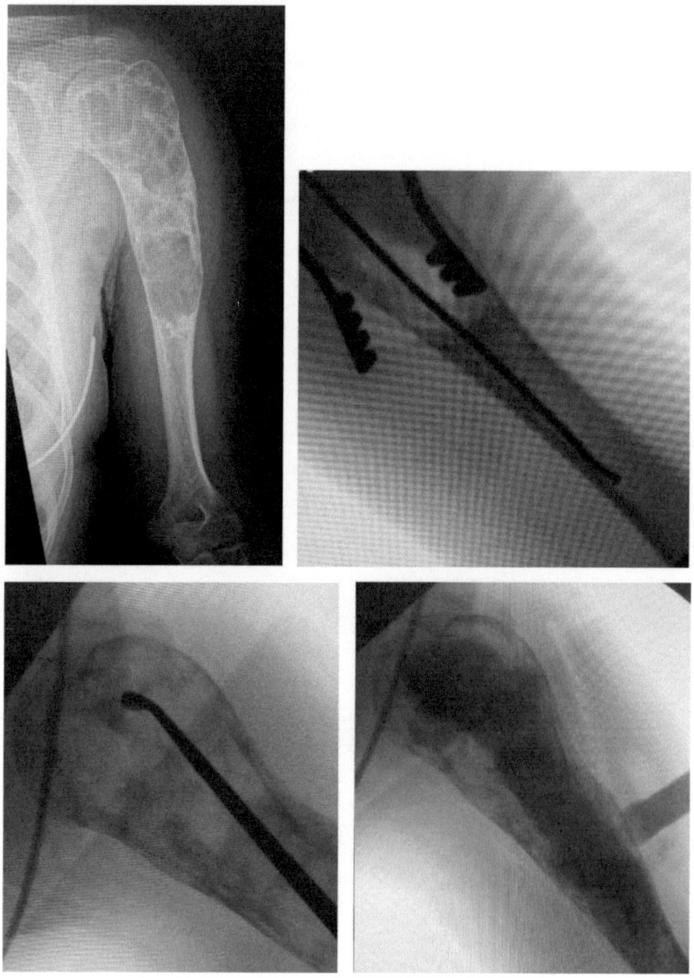

Figure 10.
Radiographic images depicting a recurrent unicameral bone cyst of the proximal humerus in a pediatric patient and its treatment. A: Unicameral bone cyst of the proximal left humerus. B: Decompression of the canal during the surgical procedure. C: Curettage of the lesion. D: Filling of the cavity with biosynthetic material composed of calcium sulfate with calcium phosphate.

5. Conclusions

Shoulder reconstruction for patients with bone tumors encompasses a diverse group of patients, diagnoses and surgical options. While most patients with primary bone tumors may be younger and more active, those with metastatic disease oftentimes are associated with an older age, worse preoperative function and worse prognosis; all factors that need to be taken into consideration in the treatment decision-making. Currently, with new advances in oncology treatments patients may benefit from longer survivals times than in the past, thus restoring the patient's function and quality of life is paramount. Ideally, an oncology orthopedic specialist ought to be included in the multidisciplinary treating team from the moment of diagnosis of bone disease.

Conflict of interest

The authors state no conflict of interest related to the writing of this chapter.

Author details

Stephanie D. Zarate and Ana C. Belzarena*
Oncology Orthopedic Service, Miami Cancer Institute, Baptist Health South Florida, Miami, Florida, United States

*Address all correspondence to: ceciliabel@baptisthealth.net

References

[1] Damron TA, Ward WG, Stewart A. Osteosarcoma, chondrosarcoma, Ewing's sarcoma: National Cancer Date Base Report. Clinical Orthopaedics and Related Research. 2007;**459**(3):40-47. DOI: 10.1097/BLO.0b013e318059b8c9

[2] Frassica FJ, Frassica DA. Evaluation and treatment of metastases to the Humerus. Clinical Orthopaedics and Related Research. 2003;**415**:S212-S218. DOI: 10.1097/01.blo.0000093052.96273.a7

[3] Trăilescu MD, Pavel AI, Pop MA, Zurbău-Anghel N, Stoica GA, Fruntelată RF, et al. Pathological fractures of humerus in children. Therapeutic and pathological considerations. Romanian Journal of Morphology and Embryology = Revue roumaine de morphologie et embryologie. 2019;**60**(3):831-840

[4] Kakhki VR, Anvari K, Sadeghi R, Mahmoudian AS, Torabian-Kakhki M. Pattern and distribution of bone metastases in common malignant tumors. Nuclear Medicine Review. 2013;**16**(2):66-69. DOI: 10.5603/NMR.2013.0037

[5] Aboulafia AJ, Kennon RE, Jelinek JS. Benign bone tumors of childhood. The Journal of the American Academy of Orthopaedic Surgeons. 1999;7:377-388

[6] Özkan EA, Göret CC, Özdemir ZT, Yanık S, Doğan M, Gönültaş A, et al. Pattern of primary tumors and tumor-like lesions of bone in children: Retrospective survey of biopsy results. International Journal of Clinical and Experimental Pathology. 2015;**8**(9):11543-11548

[7] Ruiz-Alva SK, Cortes-Cerda R, Mora-Ríos FG, Benítez-Romero A, Isunza-Ramírez A, Mejía-Rohenes LC. Tumores que producen metástasis óseas [Tumors that cause bone metastases]. Acta Ortopedica Mexicana. 2021;**35**(2):201-205

[8] Lozano Calderón SA, Garbutt C, Kim J, et al. Clinical and molecular analysis of pathologic fracture-associated osteosarcoma: MicroRNA profile is different and correlates with prognosis. Clinical Orthopaedics and Related Research. 2019;**477**(9):2114-2126. DOI: 10.1097/CORR.0000000000000867

[9] Freeman AK, Sumathi VP, Jeys L. Metastatic tumours of bone. Orthopaedics I: General Principles Surgery. 2015;**33**(1):34-39. DOI: 10.1016/j.mpsur.2014.10.005

[10] Mintz DN, Hwang S. Bone tumor imaging, then and now: Review article. HSS Journal: The Musculoskeletal Journal of Hospital for Special Surgery. 2014;**10**(3):230-239. DOI: 10.1007/s11420-014-9403-y

[11] Barnett JR, Gikas P, Gerrand C, Briggs TW, Saifuddin A. The sensitivity, specificity, and diagnostic accuracy of whole-bone MRI for identifying skip metastases in appendicular osteosarcoma and Ewing sarcoma. Skeletal Radiology. 2020;**49**(6):913-919. DOI: 10.1007/s00256-019-03364-0

[12] Gomez-Brouchet A, Mascard E, Siegfried A, de Pinieux G, Gaspar N, Bouvier C, et al. Assessment of resection margins in bone sarcoma treated by neoadjuvant chemotherapy: Literature review and guidelines of the bone group (GROUPOS) of the French sarcoma group and bone tumor study group (GSF-GETO/RESOS). Orthopaedics & Traumatology, Surgery

& Research: OTSR. 2019;**105**(4):773-780. DOI: 10.1016/j.otsr.2018.12.015

[13] Zoccali C, Attala D, Pugliese M, di Uccio AS, Baldi J. The IlluminOss® photodynamic bone stabilization system for pathological osteolyses and fractures of the humerus: Indications, advantages and limits in a series of 12 patients at 24 months of minimum follow-up. BMC Musculoskeletal Disorders. 2021;**22**(1):63. DOI: 10.1186/s12891-020-03927-6

[14] Drost L, Ganesh V, Wan BA, Raman S, Chan S, Christakis M, et al. Efficacy of postoperative radiation treatment for bone metastases in the extremities. Radiotherapy and Oncology: Journal of the European Society for Therapeutic Radiology and Oncology. 2017;**124**(1):45-48. DOI: 10.1016/j.radonc.2017.05.010

[15] Sirveaux F. Reconstruction techniques after proximal humerus tumour resection. Orthopaedics & Traumatology, Surgery & Research: OTSR. 2019;**105**(1S):S153-S164. DOI: 10.1016/j.otsr.2018.04.024

[16] Liu T, Zhang Q, Guo X, Zhang X, Li Z, Li X. Treatment and outcome of malignant bone tumors of the proximal humerus: Biological versus endoprosthetic reconstruction. BMC Musculoskeletal Disorders. 2014;**15**:69. DOI: 10.1186/1471-2474-15-69

[17] Aponte-Tinao LA, Ayerza MA, Muscolo DL, Farfalli GL. Allograft reconstruction for the treatment of musculoskeletal tumors of the upper extremity. Sarcoma. 2013;**2013**:925413

[18] Abdeen A, Hoang BH, Athanasian EA, Morris CD, Boland PJ, Healey JH. Allograft-prosthesis composite reconstruction of the proximal part of the humerus: Functional outcome and survivorship. The Journal of Bone and Joint Surgery. American Volume. 2009;**91**(10):2406-2415. DOI: 10.2106/JBJS.H.00815

[19] van de Sande MA, Dijkstra PD, Taminiau AH. Proximal humerus reconstruction after tumour resection: Biological versus endoprosthetic reconstruction. International Orthopaedics. 2011;**35**(9):1375-1380. DOI: 10.1007/s00264-010-1152-z

[20] Marulanda GA, Henderson E, Cheong D, Letson GD. Proximal and total humerus reconstruction with the use of an aortograft mesh. Clinical Orthopaedics and Related Research. 2010;**468**(11):2896-2903. DOI: 10.1007/s11999-010-1418-1

[21] Tang X, Guo W, Yang R, Tang S, Ji T. Synthetic mesh improves shoulder function after intraarticular resection and prosthetic replacement of proximal humerus. Clinical Orthopaedics and Related Research. 2015;**473**(4):1464-1471. DOI: 10.1007/s11999-015-4139-7

[22] Prantl L, Roll C, Feser D, Schreml S, Nerlich M, Mayr E, et al. Senkung der Amputationsrate bei Knochen- und Weichgewebssarkomen durch interdisziplinäres Vorgehen [Reduction of the amputation rate in bone and soft tissue sarcoma by interdisciplinary cooperation]. Handchirurgie, Mikrochirurgie, plastische Chirurgie: Organ der Deutschsprachigen Arbeitsgemeinschaft fur Handchirurgie: Organ der Deutschsprachigen Arbeitsgemeinschaft fur Mikrochirurgie der Peripheren Nerven und Gefasse: Organ der V.... 2006;**38**(3):178-184. DOI: 10.1055/s-2006-924244

[23] Voggenreiter G, Assenmacher S, Schmit-Neuerburg KP. Tikhoff-Linberg procedure for bone and soft tissue tumors of the shoulder girdle. Archives

of Surgery (Chicago, Ill: 1960). 1999;**134**(3):252-257. DOI: 10.1001/archsurg.134.3.252

[24] Tagliero AJ, Bukowski BR, Rose PS, Morrey ME, Elhassan BT, Barlow JD, et al. High incidence of complications associated with shoulder girdle reconstruction utilizing a Stryker proximal humerus cap endoprosthesis following Tikhoff-Linberg resections. International Orthopaedics. 2020;**44**(11): 2449-2455. DOI: 10.1007/s00264-020-04576-z

[25] Weisstein J. E.U. Conrad 3rd tumors and related conditions. In: Rockwood C, Matsen F, Wirth M, Lippitt S, editors. The Shoulder. 4th ed. Vol. 2. Philadelphia: Saunders Elsevier; 2009. pp. 1509-1556

[26] Schneider KN, Bröking JN, Gosheger G, Lübben T, Hardes J, Schorn D, et al. What is the implant survivorship and functional outcome after Total humeral replacement in patients with primary bone Tumors? Clinical Orthopaedics and Related Research. 2021;**479**(8):1754-1764. DOI: 10.1097/CORR.0000000000001677

[27] Lang NW, Kasparek MF, Synak L, Waldstein W, Funovics PT, Windhager R, et al. What sports activity levels are achieved in long-term survivors with modular endoprosthetic humerus reconstruction following primary bone sarcoma resection? Wiener Klinische Wochenschrift. 2021;**133**(1-2):14-20. DOI: 10.1007/s00508-020-01779-7

[28] Böhler C, Brönimann S, Kaider A, Puchner SE, Sigmund IK, Windhager R, et al. Surgical and functional outcome after Endoprosthetic reconstruction in patients with osteosarcoma of the Humerus. Scientific Reports. 2018;**8**(1):16148. DOI: 10.1038/s41598-018-34397-5

[29] Weber KL, Raymond AK. Low-grade/dedifferentiated/high-grade chondrosarcoma: A case of histological and biological progression. The Iowa Orthopaedic Journal. 2002;**22**:75-80

[30] Mik G, Arkader A, Manteghi A, Dormans JP. Results of a minimally invasive technique for treatment of unicameral bone cysts. Clinical Orthopaedics and Related Research. 2009;**467**(11):2949-2954. DOI: 10.1007/s11999-009-1008-2

[31] Deventer N, Deventer N, Gosheger G, de Vaal M, Budny T, Laufer A, et al. Chondroblastoma: Is intralesional curettage with the use of adjuvants a sufficient way of therapy? Journal of Bone Oncology. 2020;**26**:100342. DOI: 10.1016/j.jbo.2020.100342

Chapter 7

Scapular Dyskinesis

Mohammed Hegazy

Abstract

In order for correct shoulder function to occur, the scapula plays a number of responsibilities. These functions include synchronous scapular rotation during humeral motion, providing a stable basis for rotator cuff activation, and acting as a kinetic chain link. Scapular dyskinesis is defined as a change in the resting or dynamic position of the scapula. Scapular dyskinesis is a nonspecific response to a painful shoulder ailment rather than a specific response to glenohumeral pathology. Visual assessment of the scapular position at rest and during dynamic humeral motions, as well as objective posture measurements and scapular corrective techniques, is used to diagnose scapular dyskinesis. Treatment for scapular dyskinesis focuses on improving dynamic scapular stability by improving the motor control and strength of scapular stabilizers, as well as the flexibility of tight muscles and other connective tissues.

Keywords: kinetic chain, dynamic stability, scapular dyskinesis

1. Introduction

Scapular dyskinesis is a disorder characterized by altered scapular mechanics and motion, with "dys" denoting alteration and "kinesis" denoting motion [1]. Scapular dyskinesis is not always a medical word. In fact, it has been seen in both asymptomatic and symptomatic patients with shoulder girdle discomfort [2–5]. It was thought to be caused by abnormalities in scapular stabilizing muscle activation [6], injury to the long thoracic, dorsal scapular, or spinal accessory nerves, or potentially decreased pectoralis minor muscle length [7].

SICK (scapular malposition, inferior medial border prominence, coracoid pain and malposition, and dyskynesis of scapular motion) was coined by Burkhart et al. [8], who recognized the importance of scapular dyskinesis in overhead athletes complaining of shoulder pain. As a result, this term should only be used when scapular dyskinesis is clearly present.

2. Clinical features of scapular dyskinesis

The anterior and/or posterosuperior aspects of the shoulder, as well as the upper region of the lateral arm below the acromion, may be painful in the symptomatic patient with scapular dyskinesis. Pain may radiate into the lateral part of the neck along the UT or follow a radicular pattern along the upper extremity. Pain in the coracoid region due to constriction of the pectoralis minor as a result of downward tilt and lateral displacement of the coracoid is the most common presenting symptom, followed by posterosuperior scapular pain [8].

Three dyskinetic patterns were found by Kibler et al. [9]: The inferomedial border of the scapula is prominent due to an excessive posterior tilt along a horizontal axis

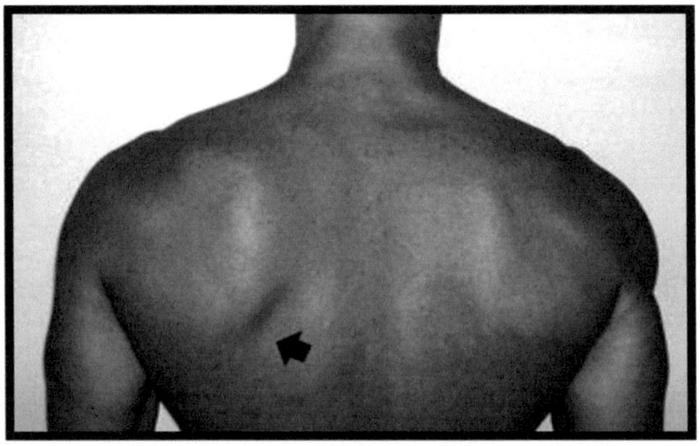

Figure 1.
Type I dyskinesis (adopted from [10]).

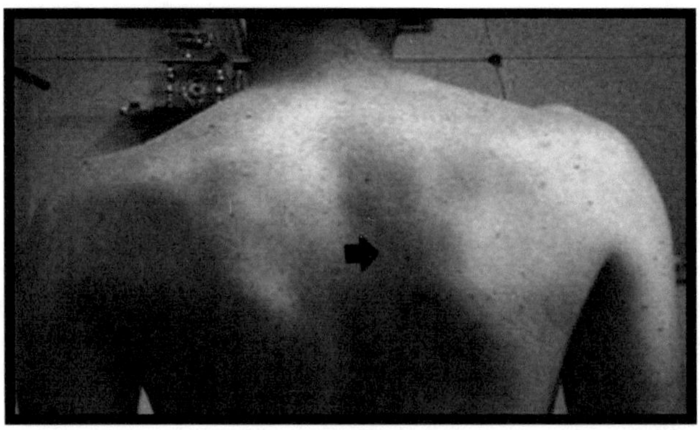

Figure 2.
Type II dyskinesis (adopted from [10]).

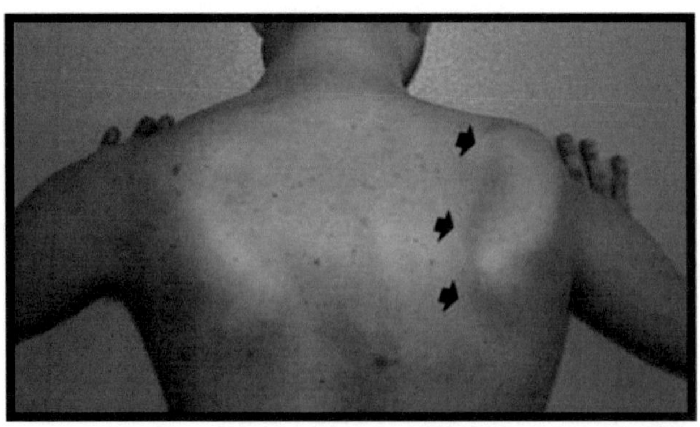

Figure 3.
Type III dyskinesis (adopted from [10]).

in the plane of the scapula; when this type is isolated, the scapula may be lower than the opposite side (**Figure 1**). Due to excessive external rotation around a vertical axis via the plane of the scapula, Type II is characterized by the prominence of its entire medial border (**Figure 2**). These types are frequently linked to superior labrum injuries. Type III is characterized by upward rotation of the scapula's superomedial border around a horizontal axis perpendicular to the plane of the scapula, resulting in abnormal superior migration of the scapula (**Figure 3**); this pattern is linked to a reduction in the acromiohumeral space and the possibility of rotator cuff injuries. The pattern of Type IV is symmetric.

3. Role of scapula

The scapula has three key functions in producing smooth, coordinated movement throughout the shoulder girdle. To sustain the glenohumeral connection and provide a stable foundation for muscle function, these tasks are intertwined. The scapula's primary function is to maintain dynamic stability and regulated motion at the glenohumeral joint. The scapula must move in sync with the moving humerus in order to keep the humeral head restricted within the glenoid during the whole range of shoulder motion [11].

Maintaining appropriate glenoid fossa alignment not only provides for ideal bony restraint, but it also aids muscular constraint by maintaining proper length tension relationships for efficient rotator cuff muscle contraction, squeezing the humeral head into the fossa [11, 12]. The scapular musculature must maintain dynamic stability while also providing regulated movement. The scapula must be protracted in a smooth fashion laterally and then anteriorly around the thoracic wall during throwing motions to allow the scapula to retain a normal positional relationship with the humerus. This motion is controlled by eccentric contraction of the medial-stabilizing musculature (mostly the rhomboids and middle trapezius), which allows part of the deceleration forces experienced during the follow-through phase to be dissipated [11].

With overhead exercises, the scapula must also rotate upward to free the acromion from the rotator cuff [13]. The scapula travels laterally in normal abduction for the first 30°–50° of abduction. As the shoulder reaches maximal elevation, the scapula rotates around a fixed axis across an arc of roughly 65° [14]. With overhead activity, the 2:1 ratio between glenohumeral abduction and scapulothoracic rotation is explained by this motion. To tilt the acromion upward and reduce the possibility of impingement and coracohumeral arch compression, upward rotation and elevation are necessary (**Figure 4**) [16].

The scapula's second function is to serve as a basis for muscular attachment. The muscles that control the position of the scapula attach to the medial border of the scapula, stabilizing it. Scapular motion is primarily controlled by this musculature through synergistic cocontractions and force couples, which are paired muscles that regulate the movement or position of a joint or a body part [17–20]. Muscles that attach along the lateral edge of the scapula perform gross motor tasks of the glenohumeral joint in addition to acting as scapular stabilizers. The rotator cuff muscles adhere to the whole surface of the scapula and are positioned so that their most efficient stabilizing activity occurs when the arm is abducted between 70° and 100° [21]. The humeral head is compressed into the socket by these muscles, which are referred to as a "compressor cuff" [20].

The scapula's third function is best described as the link in the proximal-to-distal energy transfer that enables for the ideal shoulder placement for optimal performance [16, 22–24].

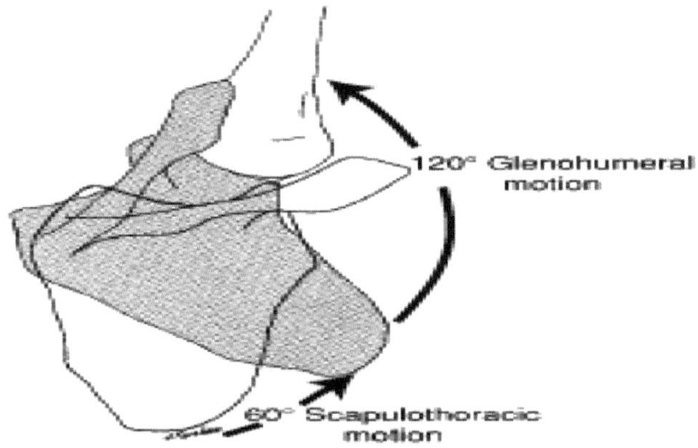

Figure 4.
Scapulohumeral rhythm (adopted from [15]).

The scapula plays a critical role in transporting enormous forces and high energy from the principal sources of force and energy, the legs and trunk, to the actual delivery mechanism of the energy and force, the arms and hands [23–25]. Forces generated in the proximal segments must be efficiently and effectively transferred via the shoulder and into the hand. The scapula provides a secure and regulated platform for these activities, allowing the entire arm to rotate as a unit around the sturdy base given by the scapulothoracic joint and the glenohumeral joints [20].

4. Scapular kinetics during arm elevation

The musculature connected to the scapula, humerus, thoracic cage, and spinal column controls the scapulothoracic articulation. During the first phase of glenohumeral elevation, the UT and lower SA operate as a force couple to cause scapular upward rotation. The LT contributes more in the intermediate phase of glenohumeral elevation, while the LT, UT, and lower SA are roughly equally active in the final phase of glenohumeral elevation. The scapular muscle is responsible for stabilizing the scapula and supporting the glenohumeral joint's base. A loss in the surrounding musculature's ability to stabilize the scapula may result in a shift in scapular position or motion. The length-tension relationship can be adjusted by changing the scapular position.

A malfunctioning rotator cuff can theoretically be caused by changes in scapular posture and scapular muscular strength [26]. The force couples' primary roles are to provide maximum congruency between the glenoid fossa and the humeral head in order to provide dynamic glenohumeral stability and maintain an ideal length-tension relationship [12, 25]. The UT and LT muscles, along with the rhomboid muscles and the SA muscle, are the appropriate force partners for scapular stabilization. The LT and SA muscles, in combination with the UT and rhomboid muscles, are the suitable force partners for acromial elevation (**Figure 5**) [20, 28].

5. Scapular kinematics during arm elevation

Normal shoulder function depends on scapular location on the thorax and control during motion. The scapula should upwardly rotate and posteriorly tilt on the

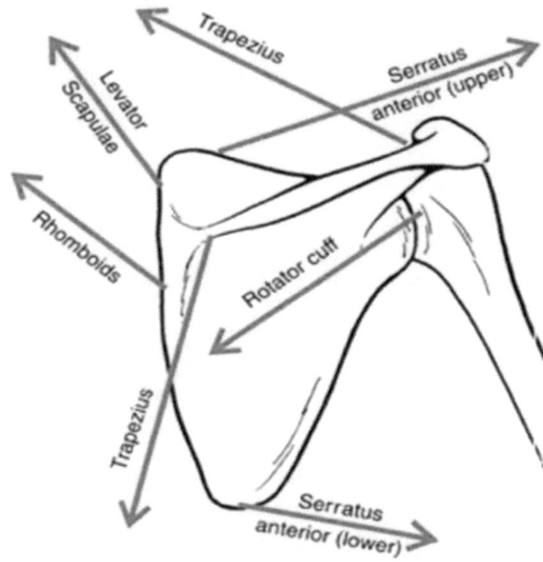

Figure 5.
Force couples of scapular stabilization (adopted from [27]).

thorax when raising the arm overhead (**Figure 6** and **Table 1**) [30]. The most common scapulothoracic motion is upward rotation. The scapula's motion in response to changes in scapular internal rotation angle is more variable between participants, investigations, elevation planes, and elevation range of motion points [30, 31]. Early in the range of arm elevation in scapular plane abduction and flexion, slight increases in scapular internal rotation may be normal. Although there is minimal data, it is generally acknowledged that end range elevation in healthy patients requires some scapulothoracic external rotation [30].

The sternoclavicular (SC) and acromioclavicular (AC) joints move together in scapulothoracic kinematics. In healthy people, substantial 3-D motions occur

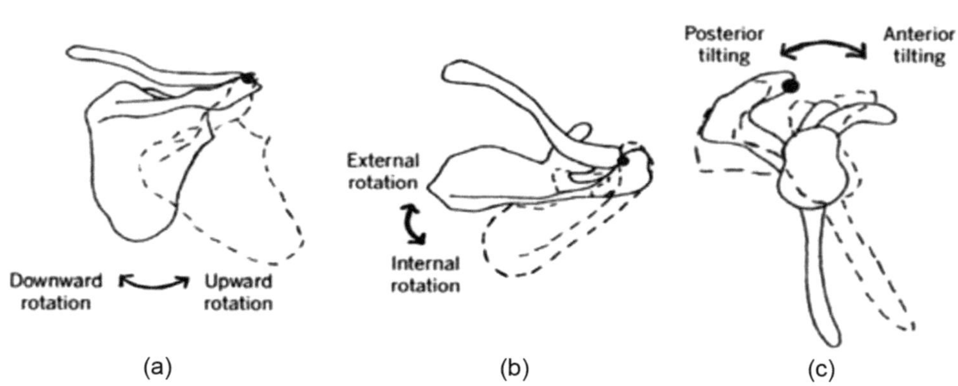

Figure 6.
Scapular motions from (a) posterior (upward/downward rotation), (b) superior (internal/external rotation), and (c) lateral (anterior/posterior tilting) views. Axes of rotation are indicated as black dots (adopted from [29]).

Motion	Healthy	Impingement or rotator cuff disease
Primary scapular motion	Upward rotation	Lesser upward rotation
Secondary scapular motion	Posterior tilting	Lesser posterior tilting
Accessory scapular motion	Variable internal/external rotation	Greater internal rotation
Presumed implications	Maximize shoulder range of motion and available subacromial space	Presumed contributory to sub acromial or internal impingement

Table 1.
Summary of scapular kinematics during arm elevation in healthy and pathologic state [29].

at both the SC and AC joints during arm elevation [30, 32, 33]. As arm elevation progresses upward, the clavicle exhibits a pattern of mild elevation and progressive retraction [30, 32]. At the AC joint, the scapula rotates upwardly, internally, and posteriorly relative to the clavicle at the same time [33]. Elevation/depression and abduction/adduction scapulothoracic "translations" have also been described in the past [33, 34]. These movements are caused by clavicular motions at the SC joint. SC elevation causes scapulothoracic elevation, and SC protraction/retraction causes abduction/adduction [33].

6. Potential biomechanical mechanisms contributing to alterations in scapular kinematics

Pain, soft tissue tightness, muscle activation or strength imbalances, muscle exhaustion, and thoracic malposture are all potential contributors to aberrant scapular kinematics (**Table 2**) [26].

6.1 Effect of muscle activity alteration on scapular kinematics

Muscle activation is the most commonly studied feature in patient populations; however, these changes in muscle activity are rarely connected to scapular kinematic changes. Significantly less SA muscle activation and greater UT activation were found in subjects with impingement or shoulder dysfunction who had less scapular upward rotation and posterior tilt as well as greater scapular elevation [35, 36].

When these findings are combined with knowledge of these muscles' ability to induce or govern scapular rotations, the lesser serratus activations may play a key role in the observed lower posterior tilt and upward rotation. Increased UT activation is likely related to greater scapula elevation by increasing clavicular elevation [37]. Scapulothoracic muscle activation timing has also been studied. In competitive freestyle swimmers with shoulder impingement, the temporal recruitment pattern of the UT, LT, and SA showed much more variability than in a control group of competitive swimmers [38].

In comparison to a control group, overhead athletes with shoulder impingement showed significantly delayed activation of the middle trapezius (MT) and

Potential biomechanical mechanisms	Associated effects
Inadequate muscle activation	Lesser scapular upward rotation and posterior tilt
Excess UT activation	Greater clavicular elevation
Pectoralis minor tightness	Greater scapular internal rotation and anterior tilt
Posterior soft tissue tightness	Greater scapular anterior tilt
Thoracic mal posture	Greater scapular internal rotation, anterior tilt and lesser scapular upward rotation

Table 2.
Potential biomechanical mechanisms contributing to scapular kinematic alterations [29].

long trapezius (LT) in response to an unexpected drop of the arm from an abducted posture [39]. The experimental production of muscular fatigue is a model for relating muscle activation patterns to changes in scapular kinematics. However, none of the studies on shoulder fatigue that have been found so far have tried to tire isolated scapulothoracic muscles, and the inability to fatigue a particular muscle or muscle group hampers interpretation of the results. One study found that after a resisted humeral external rotation fatigue treatment, scapular upward rotation, posterior tilt, and external rotation all decreased significantly. However, another study that used resisted humeral external rotation to induce shoulder fatigue reported significant increases in scapular upward rotation rather than decreases. The findings for reduced posterior tilt after fatigue were identical in direction in both studies [40, 41].

6.2 Effect of pain on scapular kinematics

The impact of pain on muscle activation patterns is likewise a mystery. Interestingly, during repetitive bilateral flexion in otherwise healthy subjects, experimentally induced pain caused by injection of hypertonic saline directly into the upper, middle, and lower divisions of the trapezius resulted in decreased UT and increased LT activation on the painful side and increased trapezius activation on the contralateral side [42].

6.3 Effect of soft tissue tightness on scapular kinematics

Another possible cause for the development of the scapulothoracic changes found in patients is soft tissue stiffness of muscles or tissues that can inhibit normal scapular motions during arm raising. Pectoralis minor and posterior shoulder stiffness have both been studied [7, 43].

6.3.1 Effect of pectoralis minor tightness on scapular kinematics

The pectoralis minor can provide scapular internal rotation, downward rotation, and anterior tilt thanks to its attachments from the coracoid process to the third to fifth ribs. Excessive active or passive tension in this muscle may prevent normal scapular upward rotation, posterior tilt, and maybe scapular external rotation from occurring during arm raising. Those with a short pectoralis minor resting length, indicative of muscular tightness, had considerably less scapular posterior tilt and more scapular internal rotation during arm elevation than those with a long pectoralis minor resting length [7].

A rounded shoulder and forward head position is a frequent postural presentation in both sedentary people and overhead sportsmen. The subacromial space shrank as the shoulder progressed from a retracted to a protracted posture, according to dynamic magnetic resonance imaging [44]. Previously, this scapula posture was linked to diminished pectoralis minor flexibility or adaptive shortening. This decreased flexibility might impact scapula posture as well as create axillary artery compression, resulting in neurovascular complaints. Because of the prolonged elongation, this postural presentation might lead to stretch weakness of the posterior scapular musculature, especially the rhomboid muscles and lower trapezius [45, 46].

6.3.2 Effect of tightness of posterior capsule on scapular kinematics

Tightness in the glenohumeral joint's posterior capsule, or posterior shoulder, has also been proposed as a mechanism for changing scapular kinematics by passively "pushing" the scapula laterally over the thorax, especially during humeral internal rotation in raised arm positions [20]. Subjects with no shoulder complaints but a glenohumeral internal rotation range-of-motion deficit on their dominant arm (indicative of posterior shoulder tightness) were compared with a control group with no such deficit in a subsequent study. The humerus was elevated 90° into both flexion and abduction postures, and scapular positioning was evaluated at end range humeral internal rotation. At end range humeral internal rotation locations, the group with less glenohumeral joint internal rotation range of motion had considerably more scapular anterior tilt [7, 43].

6.4 Effect of thoracic mal posture on scapular kinematics

Changes in scapular location have also been linked to thoracic posture. When healthy volunteers were requested to sit in a "slouched" position and raise their arm, scapular upward rotation and posterior tilt were dramatically reduced, whereas scapular internal rotation and scapular elevation were significantly increased [47]. With the arm relaxed at the side, increased scapular anterior tilt and scapular internal rotation have also been reported in women with increasing thoracic kyphosis, as well as increased scapular anterior tilt with age [48].

7. Assessment of scapular dyskinesis

The reliable and correct identification of the presence or absence of scapular position or motion abnormalities is one of the problems of the clinical diagnostic procedure in people who have shoulder pain. In one study, moderate kappa values for inter-tester and intra-tester reliability were obtained employing blinded evaluators who assessed recorded patients [9]. Another study found lower inter-rater reliability when patients were recorded and examined by therapists who were unaware of the individuals' symptom status. These dependability levels are below what is ideal for routine clinical use. Improved reliability could be achieved through direct evaluation (as opposed to film), improved training, or revision of movement category definitions [49].

The examination begins with the patient's arm at a rest. Only one, two, or all three dyskinesis patterns can be found. The stability of the SC and AC joints should be tested in the resting position, and the clavicle should be inspected for any shortening, angulation, malrotation, or hypermobility. The coracoid should be palpated to establish its position in relation to the opposite side, as well as any soreness along its medial border, where the pectoralis minor is implanted. After that, the subject is asked to raise and then drop his or her arm in the sagittal and/or scapular planes. The third stage involves watching the scapular action while lifting and lowering the arm with a 3–5 pound weight [50].

A study was conducted in asymptomatic persons and patients with shoulder discomfort to examine the reliability of the clinical assessment [2]. The patients' medial and superior scapular borders were measured as they conducted three to five arm elevation trials in the sagittal and scapular planes. The scapular motion was classified by two assessors using either the Kibler et al. [7] approach or a two-type method (yes/no). Yes, if one or more dyskinetic patterns are present, and no, if normal motion is present. To identify the presence of dyskinesis and to establish criteria validity of the two approaches, a 3-D kinematic analysis utilizing an electromagnetic tracking device was also done.

The yes/no method had a greater inter-rater agreement (79%) than the method used by Kibler et al. [51] (61%). The former strategy demonstrated a higher sensitivity (76%) and positive predictive value (100%) than the latter (74%). Multiple-plane asymmetries were detected in a substantially higher percentage of symptomatic participants (54%) than in asymptomatic subjects (14%). The researchers concluded that the yes/no technique is a good screening tool for scapular dyskinesis [10].

In contrast to these findings, Ellenbecker et al. [52] discovered that the Kibler et al. [7] technique of evaluation had a low reliability in baseball players who were videotaped performing five repetitions of scapular plane elevation while gripping a 2-pound weight. McClure et al. [50], Tate et al. [53] described a new approach for identifying scapular dyskinesis and determining its severity than Kibler et al. [7], which they called the scapular dyskinesis test. Overhead athletes were asked to do five repetitions of bilateral weighted shoulder flexion and abduction.

Dysrhythmia (premature or excessive scapular elevation or protraction, non-smooth or stuttering motion on elevation or lowering, or fast downward rotation during lowering) and/or winging are symptoms of scapular dyskinesis (medial border or inferior scapular angle posteriorly displaced from the thorax). Normal motion,

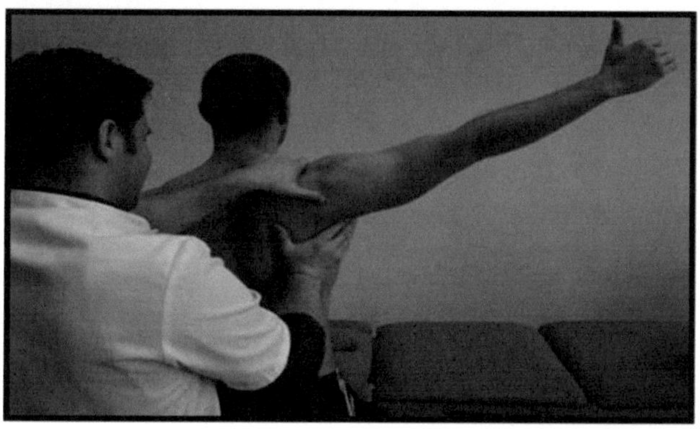

Figure 7.
Scapular assistance test (adopted from [55]).

slight abnormalities, or evident abnormalities were assigned to each scapulothoracic deviation. The raters' agreement in identifying normal or dyskinetic patients ranged from 75 to 80%. The presence of dyskinesis, on the other hand, was not linked to shoulder discomfort.

7.1 Clinical tests of scapular dyskinesis

Two corrective maneuvers can be used to confirm the kinematic changes and see if correcting them normalizes the arm motion and relieves the patient's symptoms [5, 6, 54].

7.1.1 Scapular assistance test

During humeral elevation, the examiner passively supports the scapula into upward rotation and posterior tilt with the scapular assistance test (SAT) (**Figure 7**). While the patient elevates the arm, the test is performed by pushing upward and laterally on the inferior angle of the scapula and drawing the superior aspect of the scapula posteriorly. If symptoms are relieved and motion is increased, the test is positive. The SAT helps detect the scapular contribution to impingement and rotator cuff dysfunction by increasing acromiohumeral space [56].

7.1.2 Scapular retraction/repositioning test

Tate et al. [57] described the scapular retraction/repositioning test (SRT). If a positive impingement test is found, the procedure can be redone with the scapula adjusted manually using the SRT (**Figure 8**). If symptoms are relieved and motion is increased, the test is positive. The SRT is performed by grasping the scapula with the fingers anteriorly contacting the acromioclavicular joint and the palm and thenar eminence posteriorly contacting the scapula's spine, with the forearm obliquely angled toward the inferior angle of the scapula for additional support on the medial border. The examiner's hand and forearm apply a mild push on the scapula in this manner to stimulate scapular retraction (scapular retraction test) or posterior tilting and external rotation (posterior tilting and external rotation test) (scapular repositioning test).

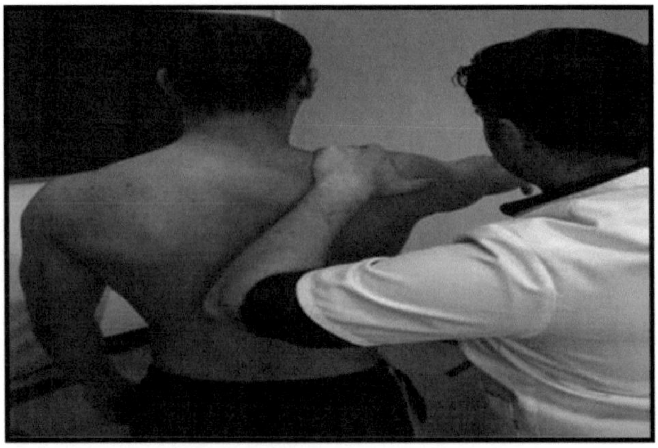

Figure 8.
Scapular retraction or repositioning test (adopted from [55]).

8. Rehabilitation of scapular dyskinesis

8.1 Stretching of pectoralis minor and posterior capsule

The pectoralis minor, posterior shoulder, and glenohumeral joint capsule are prospective candidates for stretching in individuals with scapular kinematic changes based on biomechanical variables [7, 43]. Stretching techniques for both of these tissues have been recommended. Despite the paucity of research, there have been comparisons made across procedures in terms of gains in range of motion or the potential to appropriately extend the targeted tissue [7, 58].

For posterior capsule tightness, McClure et al. [58] compared the effectiveness of a sleeper stretch, which is thought to better support the scapula, to a more standard cross-body stretch. After a 4-week stretching regimen, the passive internal rotation range of motion of asymptomatic participants was measured. Both stretching groups were also compared with a nonstretching control group. When compared with their nonstretched side, both stretching groups exhibited significant within-subject gains in range of motion. Surprisingly, only the cross-body stretch group improved much more than the control group.

In healthy subjects, the mean length change with three recommended stretches for the pectoralis minor was also compared. A unilateral self-stretch or corner stretch, as well as sitting and supine manual stretches, was among the stretches. Standing with the humerus abducted 90° and the elbow flexed 90°, the unilateral corner stretch requires placing the hand of the shoulder to stretch on the wall with the humerus abducted 90° and the elbow flexed 90°. The patient next twists their body away from the shoulder being stretched until they feel a slight strain in their pectoral muscles. The most length change was seen in the corner stretch, followed by the supine manual stretch. This shows that a corner stretch would be more successful in lengthening the pectoralis minor; however, the patients were not tracked over time in a randomized controlled trial [59].

8.2 Scapular muscle control and balance

The rehabilitation's goal is to reestablish scapular muscle control and balance [60]. The goal is to equalize the ratio between the three sections of the trapezius, that is, UT/LT and UT/MT, and activate SA, because scapular dyskinesis suggests a larger activation of the UT and a lower control of the LT, MT, and SA [10]. The push-up plus, wall slide exercises, and shoulder elevation in the scapular plane have all been demonstrated to promote SA activation, with the push-up plus causing minimal UT activation [61, 62].

In the treatment of patients with shoulder discomfort and scapular motion abnormalities, strengthening or retraining the SA muscle warrants special consideration. The SA is the only scapulothoracic muscle capable of producing all of the desired 3-D scapular rotations of upward rotation, AC joint posterior tilting, and AC joint external rotation [37, 63]; hence, this recommendation is based on its biomechanical capabilities.

The serratus anterior's position as an external rotator of the scapula may appear counterintuitive at first, given the serratus anterior's lateral line of pull around the thorax, which has led to the serratus anterior being described as causing shoulder protraction. The clavicle protracts on the thorax at the SC joint, causing this protraction. Before this secondary joint rotation can take place, the SA's line of action will pull the scapula's vertebral border and inferior angle toward the chest wall, causing external rotation of the scapula at the AC joint and stabilizing the scapula on the thorax while the clavicle protrudes [63].

A number of activities to activate the SA muscle have been recommended based on electromyographic examinations, typically in healthy participants. Push-up plus and push-up progression exercises, the dynamic embrace, supine punch, and wall sliding workouts have all been used. Supine punch and push-up plus may be advantageous for people with SIS because they increase SA muscle activation while decreasing UT muscle activation. Patients with scapular control issues may benefit from starting with supine punch exercises that stabilize the scapula against the table [48, 57, 64, 65].

The LT is another muscle that can help to support the scapula and allow for upward rotation. Shoulder flexion in the side-lying position up to 135°, prone horizontal abduction with external rotation, and shoulder external rotation in side laying have been demonstrated to elicit a beneficial ratio of lowering UT activity and raising LT activity [66].

After a brief time of teaching, Mottram et al. [67] demonstrated that normal participants can learn and repeat movements to shift the scapula into posterior tilt and upward rotation without the assistance of a physiotherapist. They discovered that all regions of the trapezius were active using a motion analysis system and surface electromyography. In two of the four exercises described by Cools et al. [66], De Mey et al. [68] discovered that conscious patient control of the scapula orientation greatly improves the activation of the three components of the trapezius without affecting the UT/MT and UT/LT ratios.

Manual scapula adjustment has been demonstrated to improve supraspinatus strength and enhance subacromial space in individuals with subacromial impingement [5, 69]. Manual scapular assistance is utilized in clinical practice to provide tactile cueing for scapula positioning in order to identify patients for whom subacromial space is a contributing factor. Shirts intended to provide tactile stimulation for good scapular placement can also be used to provide postural cueing for scapular positioning. These shirts can be worn during a rehabilitation program as well as during everyday activities (ADLs) [70].

8.3 Correction of thoracic mal posture

Thoracic posture should also be addressed in the rehabilitation of patients with shoulder impingement or rotator cuff tendinopathy, given the evidence for changed scapular kinematics with thoracic kyphosis or flexed thoracic postures [29, 47]. This includes paying attention to maintaining erect postures while performing daily activities that require arm elevation, as well as when performing shoulder workouts. Where suitable to the patient's presentation, exercises aimed at enhancing thoracic extension range of motion, strength, and endurance should be considered, keeping in mind that typical thoracic extension during arm elevation is only 10° or less [71].

Given the rhomboid's capabilities as a downward rotator of the scapula, it was suggested that excessive reliance on shoulder retraction exercises for rhomboid training as part of a postural exercise program be avoided. Another therapy option to explore is joint mobilization in the thoracic spine. In a randomized clinical trial for shoulder impingement, adding manual treatment to a supervised exercise regimen resulted in much better results than supervised exercise alone [72]. In a sample of 14 patients with primary SIS, Conroy and Hayes [73] investigated the effect of joint mobilization as part of a comprehensive therapy plan. They found that mobilization reduced pain over the course of a day as well as pain during a subacromial compression test.

8.4 Therapeutic taping

The use of therapeutic taping in the treatment of shoulder discomfort has also been studied recently. Significant changes in posture and increases in arm elevation pain-free range of motion were observed with thoracic and scapular taping designed to change posture in both participants with shoulder impingement and healthy subjects. In the impingement group, there was no significant reduction in pain during arm elevation. However, for scapular plane abduction and flexion, the point in the range of motion when increased pain was first reported was much higher (average of 15° and 16° increase in pain-free range of motion, respectively). Another study found that using taping reduced upper trapezius electromyographic activation while increasing lower trapezius electromyographic activation in participants with shoulder impingement during arm motion [74, 75].

8.5 Rhythmic stabilization exercises

Wilk and Arrigo [76] devised specific exercises to regulate the scapulothoracic joint's muscle force coupling while also stimulating proprioceptive and kinesthetic awareness to improve the scapulothoracic joint's neuromuscular control. Because of a prevalent weakness, the scapular retractors, protractors, and depressors are commonly emphasized with isolation strengthening exercises. The exercise routine for the scapula can include neuromuscular control and PNF drills. Proprioceptive awareness can be harmed as a result of macro or microtrauma; consequently, early in the rehabilitation program, the clinician should undertake drills to restore the neurosensory qualities of the joint capsule to heighten the sensory awareness of the afferent mechanoreceptors [77, 78].

8.5.1 Types of rhythmic stabilization exercises

8.5.1.1 Open kinetic chain rhythmic stabilization exercises

Manual rhythmic stabilization exercises are performed with the arm in the scapular plane at 30° of shoulder abduction, starting with the internal and external rotators. A cocontraction of the internal and external rotators is enabled by varying manual input, which necessitates the patient's isometric stability. These stability drills can also be done with the arm at around 100° of elevation and 10° of horizontal abduction. Because of the combined centralized resultant force vectors of both the rotator cuff and deltoid musculature that induce humeral head compression, this "balanced position" is a favorable beginning point [14, 79].

8.5.1.2 Closed kinetic chain rhythmic stabilization exercises

Proprioceptive drills are used to advance closed kinetic chain workouts. Advanced weight-shifting drills include a table push-up on a ball or on an unstable surface. Completing a push-up exercise on an unstable or modified surface has been demonstrated to create higher upper trapezius, middle trapezius, and serratus anterior activation in overhead throwing athletes with impingement than performing a regular push-up exercise. While the patient's hand is on a little ball and the physician performs perturbation drills on the patient's arm, wall stabilizations are conducted [15].

9. Conclusions

Scapular dyskinesis is a multifactorial disorder characterized by changes in scapular kinematics during position and motion. Scapular dyskinesis should be assessed on both static and dynamic levels, with treatment focusing on scapula motor control and increasing the force couple around the scapula to improve shoulder dynamic stability.

Acknowledgements

I thank ALLAH for all things in my life. My thanks to my parents, my wife, and my dear sons.

Notes/thanks/other declarations

Thanks to ALLAH for helping me to finish this work.

Acronyms and abbreviations

UT	upper trapezius
MT	middle trapezius
LT	lower trapezius
SA	serratus anterior

Author details

Mohammed Hegazy[1,2]

1 Faculty of Physical Therapy, Cairo University, Giza, Egypt

2 Faculty of Allied of Medical Sciences, Isra University, Amman, Jordan

*Address all correspondence to: mohamed.mostafa@pt.cu.edu.eg; mohammed.hegazy@iu.edu.jo

References

[1] Kibler WB, Sciascia A. Current concepts: Scapular dyskinesis. British Journal of Sports Medicine. 2010;**44**(5):330-335

[2] Uhl TL, Kibler WB, Gecewich B, Tripp BL. Evaluation of clinical assessment methods for scapular dyskinesis. Arthroscopy. 2009;**25**(11):1240-1248

[3] Silva RT, Hartmann LG, de Souza Laurino CF. Clinical and ultrasonographic correlation between scapular dyskinesia and subacromial space measurement among junior elite tennis players. British Journal of Sports Medicine. 2010;**44**(6):407-410

[4] Juul-Kristensen B, Hilt K, Enoch F, Remvig L, Sjøgaard G. Scapular dyskinesis in trapezius myalgia and intraexaminer reproducibility of clinical tests. Physiotherapy Theory and Practice. 2011;**27**(7):492-502

[5] Seitz AL, McClure PW, Lynch SS, Ketchum JM, Michener LA. Effects of scapular dyskinesis and scapular assistance test on subacromial space during static arm elevation. Journal of Shoulder and Elbow Surgery. 2012;**21**(5):631-640

[6] Kibler WB, McMullen J. Scapular dyskinesis and its relation to shoulder pain. The Journal of the American Academy of Orthopaedic Surgeons. 2003;**11**(2):142-151

[7] Borstad JD, Ludewig PM. The effect of long versus short pectoralis minor resting length on scapular kinematics in healthy individuals. The Journal of Orthopaedic and Sports Physical Therapy. 2005;**35**(4):227-238

[8] Burkhart SS, Morgan CD, Kibler WB. The disabled throwing shoulder: Spectrum of pathology part III: The SICK scapula, scapular dyskinesis, the kinetic chain, and rehabilitation. Arthroscopy. 2003;**19**(6):641-661

[9] Kibler WB, Uhl TL, Maddux JW, Brooks P, Zeller B, McMullen J. Quantitative clinical evaluation of scapular dysfunction: A reliability study. Journal of Shoulder and Elbow Surgery. 2002;**11**:11550-11556

[10] Postacchini R, Carbone S. Scapular dyskinesis: Diagnosis and treatment. OA Musculoskeletal Medicine. 2013;**1**(2):20

[11] Pink M, Perry J. Biomechanics. In: Jobe FW, editor. Operative Techniques in Upper Extremity Sports Injuries. St Louis, MO: Mosby; 1996. pp. 109-123

[12] Kamkar A, Irrgang JJ, Whitney SL. Nonoperative management of secondary shoulder impingement syndrome. The Journal of Orthopaedic and Sports Physical Therapy. 1993;**17**:212-224

[13] Kibler WB. Evaluation of sports demands as a diagnostic tool in shoulder disorders. In: Matsen FA, Fu F, Hawkins RJ, editors. The Shoulder: A Balance of Mobility and Stability. Rosemont, IL: American Academy of Orthopaedic Surgeons; 1993. pp. 379-395

[14] Poppen NK, Walker PS. Normal and abnormal motion of the shoulder. Journal of Bone and Joint Surgery. 1976;**58**:195-201

[15] Levangie, P. K., & Norkin, C. C. (2011). *Joint structure and function: a comprehensive analysis*. FA Davis

[16] Kennedy K. Rehabilitation of the unstable shoulder. Operative Techniques in Sports Medicine. 1993;**1**:311-324

[17] Bagg SD, Forrest WJ. Electromyographic study of the scapular rotators during arm abduction in the scapular plane. American Journal of Physical Medicine. 1986;**65**:111-124

[18] DiGiovine NM, Jobe FW, Pink M, Perry J. An electromyographic analysis of the upper extremity in pitching. Journal of Shoulder and Elbow Surgery. 1992;**1**:15-25

[19] Moseley JB Jr, Jobe FW, Pink M, Perry J, Tibone JE. EMG analysis of the scapular muscles during a shoulder rehabilitation program. The American Journal of Sports Medicine. 1992;**20**:128-134

[20] Kibler WB. The role of the scapula in athletic shoulder function. American Journal of Sports Medicine. 1998;**26**:325-337

[21] Bak K, Faunl P. Clinical findings in competitive swimmers with shoulder pain. The American Journal of Sports Medicine. 1997;**25**:254-260

[22] Fleisig GS, Dillman CJ, Andrews JR. Biomechanics of the shoulder during throwing. In: Andrews JR, Wilk KE, editors. The Athlete's Shoulder. New York, NY: Churchill Livingstone; 1994. pp. 355-368

[23] Elliott BC, Marshall R, Noffal G. Contributions of upper limb segmentrotations during the power serve in tennis. Journal of Applied Biomechanics. 1995;**11**:433-442

[24] Kibler WB. Biomechanical analysis of the shoulder during tennis activities. Clinical Journal of Sport Medicine. 1995;**14**:79-85

[25] Kibler WB. Role of the scapula in the overhead throwing motion. Contemporary Orthopaedics. 1991;**22**:525-532

[26] Michener LA, McClure PW, Karduna AR. Anatomical and biomechanical mechanisms of subacromial impingement syndrome. Clinical Biomechanics. 2003;**18**(5):369-379

[27] Hamill, J., & Knutzen, K. Foundations of human movement & functional anatomy. In *Biomechanical Basis of Human Movement*. Wolters Kluwer Health/Lippincott Williams & Wilkins. 2009. pp. 3-25

[28] Peat M. Functional anatomy of the shoulder complex. Physical Therapy. 1986;**66**:1855-1865

[29] Van der Helm FC, Pronk GM. Three-dimensional recording and description of motions of the shoulder mechanism. Journal of Biomechanical Engineering. 1995;**117**:27-40

[30] McClure PW, Michener LA, Sennett BJ, Karduna AR. Direct 3-dimensional measurement of scapular kinematics during dynamic movements in vivo. Journal of Shoulder and Elbow Surgery. 2001:269-277

[31] Borstad JD, Ludewig PM. Comparison of scapular kinematics between elevation and lowering of the arm in the scapular plane. Clinical Biomechanics (Bristol, Avon). 2002;**17**:650-665

[32] Ludewig PM, Behrens SA, Meyer SM, Spoden SM, Wilson LA. Three-dimensional clavicular motion during arm elevation: Reliability and descriptive data. The Journal of Orthopaedic and Sports Physical Therapy. 2004:140-149

[33] Teece RM, Lunden JB, Lloyd AS, Kaiser AP, Cieminski CJ, Ludewig PM. Three-dimensional acromioclavicular joint motions during elevation of the arm. Journal of Orthopaedic & Sports Physical Therapy. 2008;**38**:181-190

[34] Lukaseiwicz AC, McClure P, Michener L, Pratt N, Sennett B.

Comparison of 3 dimensional scapular position and orientation between subjects with and without shoulder impingement. Journal of Orthopaedic and Sports Physical Therapy. 1999;**29**(10):574-583

[35] Ludewig PM, Cook TM. Alterations in shoulder kinematics and associated muscle activity in people with symptoms of shoulder impingement. Physical Therapy. 2000;**80**(3):276-291

[36] Lin JJ, Hanten WP, Olson SL. Functional activity characteristics of individuals with shoulder dysfunctions. Journal of Electromyography and Kinesiology. 2005;**15**:576-586

[37] Fey AJ, Dorn CS, Busch BP, Laux LA, Hassett DR, Ludewig PM. Potential torque capabilities of the trapezius [abstract]. The Journal of Orthopaedic and Sports Physical Therapy. 2007;**37**:A44-A45

[38] Wadsworth DJ, Bullock-Saxton JE. Recruitment patterns of the scapular rotator muscles in freestyle swimmers with subacromial impingement. International Journal of Sports Medicine. 1997;**18**:618-624

[39] Cools AM, Witvrouw EE, Declercq GA, Danneels LA, Cambier DC. Scapular muscle recruitment patterns: Trapezius muscle latency with and without impingement symptoms. The American Journal of Sports Medicine. 2003;**31**(4):542-549

[40] Tsai NT, McClure PW, Karduna AR. Effects of muscle fatigue on 3-dimensional scapular kinematics. Archives of Physical Medicine and Rehabilitation. 2003;**84**:1000-1005

[41] Ebaugh DD, McClure PW, Karduna AR. Scapulothoracic and glenohumeral kinematics following an external rotation fatigue protocol. The Journal of Orthopaedic and Sports Physical Therapy. 2006;**36**:557-571

[42] Falla D, Farina D, Graven-Nielsen T. Experimental muscle pain results in reorganization of coordination among trapezius muscle subdivisions during repetitive shoulder flexion. Experimental Brain Research. 2007;**178**:385-393

[43] Borich MR, Bright JM, Lorello DJ, Cieminski CJ, Buisman T, Ludewig PM. Scapular angular positioning at end range internal rotation in cases of glenohumeral internal rotation deficit. The Journal of Orthopaedic and Sports Physical Therapy. 2006:926-934

[44] Solem-Bertoft E, Thuomas KA, Westerberg CE. The influence of scapular retraction and protraction on the width of the subacromial space. An MRI study. Clinical Orthopaedics and Related Research. 1993;**296**:99-103

[45] Rohrer MJ, Cardullo PA, Pappas AM, Phillips DA, Wheeler HB. Axillary artery compression and thrombosis throwing athletes. Journal of Vascular Surgery. 1990;**11**(6):761-768

[46] Sotta RP. Vascular problems in the proximal upper extremity. Clinics in Sports Medicine. 1990;**9**(2):379-388

[47] Kebaetse M, McClure P, Pratt NA. Thoracic position effect on shoulder range of motion, strength, and three-dimensional scapular kinematics. Archives of Physical Medicine and Rehabilitation. 1999;**80**:945-950

[48] Decker MJ, Hintermeister RA, Faber KJ, Hawkins RJ. Serratus anterior muscle activity during selected rehabilitation exercises. The American Journal of Sports Medicine. 1999;**27**:784-791

[49] Hickey BW, Milosavljevic S, Bell ML, Milburn PD. Accuracy and reliability of observational motion analysis in identifying shoulder symptoms. Manual Therapy. 2007:263-270

[50] McClure PW, Tate AR, Kareha S, Irwin D, Zlupko E. A clinical method for identifying scapular dyskinesis, part 1: Reliability. Journal of Athletic Training. 2009;**44**(2):160-164

[51] Kibler, W. B., Uhl, T. L., Maddux, J. W., Brooks, P. V., Zeller, B., & McMullen, J. Qualitative clinical evaluation of scapular dysfunction: a reliability study. *Journal of shoulder and elbow surgery*. 2002;**11**(6):550-556

[52] Ellenbecker TS, Kibler WB, Bailie DS, Caplinger R, Davis GJ, Riemann BL. Reliability of scapular classification in examination of professional baseball players. Clinical Orthopaedics and Related Research. 2012;**470**(6):1540-1544

[53] Tate AR, McClure P, Kareha S, Irwin D, Barbe MF. A clinical method for identifying scapular dyskinesis, part 2: Validity. Journal of Athletic Training. 2009;**44**(2):165-173

[54] Jobe FW, Moynes DR. Delineation of diagnostic criteria and a rehabilitation program for rotator cuff injuries. The American Journal of Sports Medicine. 1982;**10**(6):336-339

[55] Struyf, F., Nijs, J., Mottram, S., Roussel, N. A., Cools, A. M., & Meeusen, R. Clinical assessment of the scapula: a review of the literature. *British journal of sports medicine*. 2014;**48**(11):883-890

[56] Tate AR, McClure PW, Kareha S, Irwin D. Effect of the scapula reposition test on shoulderimpingement symptoms and elevation strength in overhead athletes. The Journal of Orthopaedic and Sports Physical Therapy. 2008;**38**:4-11

[57] Rubin BD, Kibler WB. Fundamental principles of shoulder rehabilitation: Conservative to postoperative management. Arthroscopy. 2002;**18** (9 Suppl. 2):29-39

[58] Borstad JD, Ludewig PM. Comparison of three stretches for the pectoralis minormuscle. Journal of Shoulder and Elbow Surgery. 2006;**15**:324-330

[59] Culham E, Peat M. Functional anatomy of the shoulder complex. The Journal of Orthopaedic and Sports Physical Therapy. 1993;**18**:342-350

[60] Hardwick DH, Beebe JA, McDonnell MK, Lang CE. A comparison of serratus anterior muscle activation during a wall slide exercise and other traditional exercises. The Journal of Orthopaedic and Sports Physical Therapy. 2006;**36**(12):903-910

[61] Cricchio M, Frazer C. Scapulothoracic and scapulohumeral exercises: A narrative review of electromyographic studies. Journal of Hand Therapy. 2011;**24**(4):322-333

[62] Van der Helm FC. Analysis of the kinematic and dynamic behavior of the shoulder mechanism. Journal of Biomechanics. 1994;**27**:527-550

[63] Lear LJ, Gross MT. An electromyographical analysis of the scapular stabilizing synergists during a push-up progression. The Journal of Orthopaedic and Sports Physical Therapy. 1998;**28**:146-157

[64] Ludewig PM, Hoff MS, Osowski EE, Meschke SA, Rundquist PJ. Relative balance of serratus anterior and upper trapezius muscle activity during push-up exercises. The American Journal of Sports Medicine. 2004b;**32**:484-493

[65] Cools AM, Dewitte V, Lanszweert F, Notebaert D, Roets A, Soetens B. Rehabilitation of scapular muscle balance: Which exercises to prescribe? The American Journal of Sports Medicine. 2007;**35**(10):1744-1751

[66] Mottram SL, Woledge RC, Morrissey D. Motion analysis study of a scapular orientation exercise and subjects' ability to learn the exercise. Manual Therapy. 2009;**14**(1):13-18

[67] De Mey K, Danneels LA, Cagnie B, Huyghe L, Seyns E, Cools AM. Conscious correction of scapular orientation in overhead athletes performing selected shoulder rehabilitation exercises: The effect on trapezius muscle activation measured by surface electromyography. The Journal of Orthopaedic and Sports Physical Therapy. 2013;**43**(1):3-10

[68] Kibler WB, Sciascia A, Dome D. Evaluation of apparent and absolute supraspinatus strength in patients with shoulder injury using the scapular retraction test. American Journal of Sports Medicine. 2006;**34**:1643-1647

[69] Escamilla RF, Hooks TR, Wilk KE. Optimal management of shoulder impingement syndrome. Open Access Journal of Sports Medicine. 2014;**5**:13

[70] McClure PW, Balaicuis J, Heiland D, Broersma ME, Thorndike CK, Wood A. A randomized controlled comparison of stretching procedures for posterior shoulder tightness. Journal of Orthopaedic & Sports Physical Therapy. 2007;**37**(3):108-114

[71] Ludewig PM, Reynolds JR. The association of scapular kinematics and glenohumeral joint pathologies. Journal of Orthopaedic and Sports Physical Therapy. 2009;**39**(2):90-104

[72] Conory DE, Hayes KW. The effect of joint mobilization as a component of comprehensive treatment for primary shoulder impingement syndrome. Journal of Orthopaedic & Sports Physical Therapy. 1998;**28**:3-14

[73] Lewis JS, Wright C, Green A. Subacromial impingement syndrome: The effect of changing posture on shoulder range of movement. The Journal of Orthopaedic and Sports Physical Therapy. 2005:72-87

[74] Selkowitz DM, Chaney C, Stuckey SJ, Vlad G. The effects of scapular taping on the surface electromyographic signal amplitude of shoulder girdle muscles during upper extremity elevation in individuals with suspected shoulder impingement syndrome. The Journal of Orthopaedic and Sports Physical Therapy. 2007;**37**:694-702

[75] Wilk KE, Arrigo CA. An integrated approach to upper extremity exercises. Orthopaedic Physical Therapy Clinics of North America. 1992;**1**:337-360

[76] Lephart SM, Warner JJ, Borsa PA, Fu FH. Proprioception of the shoulder joint in healthy, unstable, and surgically repaired shoulders. Journal of Shoulder and Elbow Surgery. 1994;**3**(6):371-380

[77] Lephart SM, Pincivero DM, Giraldo JL, Fu FH. The role of proprioception in the management and rehabilitation of athletic injuries. The American Journal of Sports Medicine. 1997;**25**(1):130-137

[78] Walker PS, Poppen NK. Biomechanics of the shoulder joint during abduction in the plane of the scapula [proceedings]. Bulletin of the Hospital for Joint Diseases. 1977;**38**(2):107-111

[79] Tucker WS, Armstrong CW, Gribble PA, Timmons MK, Yeasting RA. Scapular muscle activity in overhead athletes with symptoms of secondary shoulder impingement during closed chain exercises. Archives of Physical Medicine and Rehabilitation. 2010;**91**(4):550-556